Surviving Prostate Cancer
A Personal Journey and Second Opinion

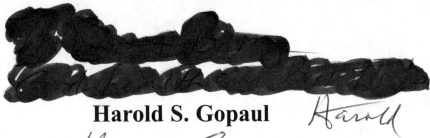

Harold S. Gopaul

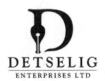

Detselig Enterprises Ltd.
Calgary, Alberta, Canada

Library and Archives Canada Cataloguing in Publication

Gopaul, Harold S

Surviving prostate cancer : a personal journey & second opinion / Harold S. Gopaul.

Includes bibliographical references. ISBN-13: 978-1-55059-323-5 ISBN-10: 1-55059-323-4

1. Prostate – Cancer – Popular works. I. Title.

RC280.P7G665 2006   616.99'463   C2006-902513-4

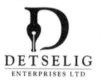

Detselig Enterprises Ltd.

210, 1220 Kensington Road NW
Calgary, Alberta
T2N 3P5

Phone: (403) 283-0900
Fax: (403) 283-6947
Email: temeron@telusplanet.net
Website: www.temerondetselig.com

We acknowledge the financial support of the Government of Canada through the Book Publishing Industry Development Program (BPIDP) for our publishing activities.

We also acknowledge the support of the Alberta Foundation for the Arts for our publishing program.

Alberta
Foundation
for the Arts

1-55059-323-4   978-1-55059-323-5 SAN 113-0234 Printed in Canada

This book is dedicated to the men, their spouses, partners and families of Prostate Support Groups from Newfoundland to Vancouver Island.

A Note to the Reader

The information presented in this book is not intended to replace the advice of doctors and other trained health professionals. No medical advice is contained in this book and it is important to consult with your doctor; furthermore, the information does not provide a complete guide on prevention, detection, diagnosis and treatment options for prostate cancer. The contents represent my opinion, personal experiences and the research cited in the literature. The author and publisher strongly advise undiagnosed men and prostate cancer patients to obtain all matters regarding your health from your primary care physician, urologist or oncologist who are familiar with your condition and medical history. The author or publisher is not liable for any loss, damage or injury as a consequence of the information presented in this book.

While every effort was made to check the accuracy of telephone numbers, Internet addresses and citations at the time of publication, neither the author nor the publisher assumes any responsibility for any inaccuracies, errors or omissions.

About the Author:

Harold Gopaul taught biology and worked in British Columbia, West Africa and in the Middle East. He is a former Editor of the British Columbia Science Teachers' journal, the Catalyst, and the pioneering Editor of the Newsletter of the Vancouver Prostate Support Group. He has authored and co-authored three books. Harold Gopaul is the recipient of the Distinguished Service Award of the B.C. Science Teachers' Association. In 1985, he was presented with an Outstanding Biology Teacher Award by the U.S. National Association of Biology Teachers. He is a prostate cancer survivor and a member of the Vancouver and Coquitlam Prostate Support and Awareness Groups.

Acknowledgments

I would like to thank my general practitioner who has been diligently treating and advising me for the past 25 years with compassion and professional care. Thanks also to my urologist who was responsible for confirming my diagnosis of having prostate cancer by first doing a biopsy and later performed nerve-sparing retropubic radical prostatectomy about twelve years ago. I would like to pay tribute to the men and women of the *Coquitlam and Vancouver Prostate Support and Awareness Groups in British Columbia,* for their continuing efforts in promoting prostate cancer awareness; to Len Gross for his tireless work as coordinator of the Vancouver PSA group for over 12 years. I greatly appreciated the staff at the Vancouver Cancer Agency Library who provided me with free access to do my research. I would like to express my sincere thanks also to the National Institutes of Health and the National Cancer Institute in the United States for providing me with graphics and other materials, without which this book will not be complete. The Canadian Prostate Cancer Network, a voice of prostate cancer in Canada, continues to be very supportive in making the Canadian public and patients more aware about prostate cancer.

I am very grateful to the reviewers of the manuscript: First, I owe a great deal of thanks to Dr. Scott Tyldesley, a radiation oncologist at the Vancouver Cancer Clinic, for his constructive criticisms and support; to Dr. Hal Gunn, the Director of The Centre for Integrated Healing in Vancouver, for his professional advice and review of materials pertaining to the work at the Centre; to Dr. Joe McGinnis, a physician, for his encouragement and support; to Craig Asmundson, Dan Cohen, Gordon Clay, and Norm Sherling who have been treated for prostate cancer and are actively involved with Prostate Support Groups in British Columbia, for their valuable observations and suggestions. Last but not least, I owe a great deal to my family for their encouragement and support before, during and after my treatment for prostate cancer.

Harold Gopaul, B.Sc., M.A., Dip. Ed.

Contents

Preface

I wish that I had known more about prostate cancer and its treatment before I was first diagnosed almost twelve years ago. I would have considered a different hormonal therapy prior to having my surgery. I would have also consulted with a radiation oncologist even though I felt that I had made the right decision for my treatment. My prostate specific antigen test or PSA was a surprising 0.2 microgram per litre; my Gleason score was 5 (2+3 grades) with mostly well differentiated tissue, and I was in very good health at an age of 57 years. Surgery was my best option since my cancer was confined to the prostate and given my Gleason score and PSA. My physician discovered a palpable tumour through an initial digital rectal examination that was part of my an annual physical examination. Malignancy or extent of my cancer involved 10 percent of the gland. I am sure that a liaison with a prostate support group immediately following my diagnosis would have also been helpful in alleviating some of my concerns and anxieties.

The information presented in this book was researched using the literature from eminent medical and scientific journals, medical books, selected websites and supporting links on prostate cancer which I have listed at the end of this book. Having an academic biology background and being touched with prostate cancer, I believe that I am able to share with you the updated research and second opinions presented in the literature from the 1990s and up to 2006, the time of writing, while incorporating my experiences in this personal journey. Wherever possible throughout the text I have presented some of my concerns and the problems encountered before and after my treatment. I hope this information will be useful, and especially to undiagnosed men, their spouses, partners and family members. In my opinion, men and women need to educate themselves more on health issues; this publication provides an opportunity to the reader to become more aware about prostate cancer and to make educated decisions on prevention, detection and treatment options.

By conducting extensive research of the literature, including my long time association with the Vancouver Prostate Support and Awareness Group, the need to share my experiences with having prostate cancer and its treatment, encouraged me to write this book. I am aware of the fears, anxieties, concerns as well as some misunderstanding men have about this disease. I believe that it is to your advantage to gain some understanding about prostate cancer or any life-threatening illness, even for the undiagnosed. It is important to keep a personal medical file of any tests that you have taken so as to monitor your progress or condition over the years. Do not hesitate to ask your doctor questions about your physical or mental health or of the results of any tests that you have taken. It may be necessary to discuss your medical concerns with close relatives and friends, including the men in a prostate cancer support group. Reading the information in this book will allow you to make sensible decisions about your own health well before you visit your physician. You may also wish to obtain a second opinion on any treatment option offered, be it hormonal therapy, radical prostatectomy or surgery, external beam radiation, brachytherapy, or for an objectified active surveillance, formerly known as watchful waiting. I have provided access to a number of second opinions throughout this book and encourage the reader to take charge of his or her own health.

The incidence of prostate cancer is apparently increasing in Canada and the United States mainly due to earlier detection of the disease; it is the most commonly diagnosed internal cancer among men. One in seven Canadian men will develop clinically significant prostate during his lifetime and one in 26 men will die from it. About 20 percent of men who are diagnosed with prostate cancer die from it, so being diagnosed is not a death sentence; cancer is curable and some types are preventable. Earlier patient detection, diagnosis and modern therapies of treating prostate cancer, in my opinion, would lower the mortality rate. Prostate cancer is the second leading cause of cancer mortality among males, with lung cancer still being the biggest cancer killer for both sexes. In my opinion, men over 40 years of age should have a digital rectal examination (DRE) when undergoing a physical examination and a follow up with the PSA serum blood test. Men whose immediate relatives were diagnosed with prostate cancer and African-Canadian men should be tested earlier. Men in recent years are becoming more concerned about their health and are consulting with their doctors on a more regular basis. Guidelines on PSA screening from various sources are presented in Chapters 5 and 11. The PSA test as a valuable diagnostic tool to evaluate a man's prostate condition is discussed in detail in Chapter 5. More specific prostate cancer markers are becoming available that would reduce the need for a biopsy.

Having been diagnosed with prostate cancer, I wanted to know as much as possible about this disease that became part of my ongoing therapy. Mahatma Gandhi once said: "It is knowledge that ultimately gives salvation." When I was first diagnosed, I was spending more time reading about prostate cancer from as many sources I could get my hands on rather than preparing my teaching material. Some physicians hold conflicting views on early prostate cancer detection, screening, the way in which the PSA test is being interpreted and on treatment options. By reading this book, I believe the reader will be able to make sound decisions when consulting with primary care physicians and medical specialists. Every effort was made to check the accuracy of the materials presented in the references cited. As a cautionary note to the reader, the information presented in this book on detection, diagnosis and treatment options should be used as a guide and is not intended to replace the expert advice of doctors and other trained health professionals; furthermore, the contents represent my personal experiences and opinions, and are based upon the research cited in the literature listed in the text.

Chapter 1

The Biology of the Prostate

By reading this chapter you will learn:
- The importance of the prostate gland.
- The main function of the reproductive system.
- How the prostate gland continues to change as a man ages.
- The endocrine system and its interactions in the human male.
- Why is testosterone important?
- The role of androgens influencing the prostate gland.
- A genetic link to prostate cancer.

The Prostate Gland and Endocrine Activity

I should confess that as a high school biology teacher my knowledge of the prostate gland was limited to the reproductive system of small mammals and the maintenance of the activity of sperm cells as its main function. I also paid little attention to this gland in the dissection of preserved rats, cats and fetal pigs, only that my students had to know its location and basic role in relation to the reproductive system. I never realized that this gland would prove to be such a grave problem for me in later life. The majority of men still do not understand the role of the prostate gland and some surprisingly do not even know where it is located in the body. Urologist Stephen Rous commented that there is more misunderstanding, more concern, and greater anxieties about the prostate gland than any other part of the male reproductive system. Urologist Peter Scardino writing in his book, *Prostate Cancer,* said that he was once being discouraged from focusing on prostate cancer as a specialty by his professors "because prostate cancer was far too complex." In a survey conducted in the United States some years ago, men were asked questions about their knowledge of the prostate; nearly 50 percent did not know where the prostate was located and another 60 percent did not know its purpose. I am certain that, if a survey were conducted today, there would be more favourable results in Canada and in the U.S. as many men have become more knowledgeable about prostate diseases.

Having taught biology for 35 years and being touched with prostate cancer, I believe that I am able to discuss some of the research materials dealing with prostate cancer, its treatment options and provide personal experiences of having this disease. I will use some biological and health related terms throughout the text and have included a **glossary** at the end to clarify most of the key words that may perhaps be confusing. The name **prostate** is derived from the Greek language meaning "before" and "to stand" because it stands before the bladder. It is an **exocrine** gland primarily because it secretes important fluids that mix with sperm cells during a man's ejaculation. The prostate gland is under the influence of the male sex hormone **testosterone** and produces its own hormone, **dihydrotestosterone** (DHT), for its function. A hormone is a chemical messenger produced in one part of the body that controls the function or activity of other parts in the individual. Testosterone is the male hormone secreted from **Leydig cells** in the testes and under the influence of **luteinizing hormone** (LH) from the **pituitary gland** in the brain. Another hormone of importance and secreted from the **hypothalamus** of the brain is **luteinizing hormone releasing hormone** (LHRH) which regulates and influences the production of LH. Thus, LHRH indirectly regulates the secretion of testosterone. The hypothalamus is connected to and located above the pituitary gland in the mid-ventral region of the brain. Chapter 9 reviews hormonal interactions and therapy.

So what does the prostate do? The prostate converts testosterone into a major biological metabolite, the hormone **dihydrotestosterone** (DHT) which is "almost as essential to the prostate as oxygen is to most cells," according to Drs. Farnsworth and Ablin. Testosterone is metabolized into DHT with the help of an enzyme known as **5-alpha-reductase.** DHT binds to certain receptors in the prostate gland that subsequently releases a number of growth factors. It is the action of DHT that activates the growth of benign prostate tumours. It is interesting to note that one metabolite of DHT is referred to as 3-alpha-androstanediol glucuronide and is the more active form of testosterone in the prostate gland, as explained in a study by Dr. Cheng and investigators. Researchers are still unaware how cancer develops in the prostate, but the role of hormones, inheritance factors, dietary intake or lack of, and certain growth factors are collectively implicated. Only about two percent to three percent of the circulating body testosterone is free (not bound to a protein) and that active free component is used to target the prostate gland. Dr. Gann and collaborators investigated the blood levels of hormones in men with and without prostate cancer. They found that high levels of circulating testosterone and low levels of sex hormone-binding globulin are associated with increased risk of prostate cancer. They noted that circulating DHT and 3alpha-androstanediol glucuronide do not appear to be strongly related to prostate cancer risk.

Overview of the Prostate Gland

The prostate is a large male accessory reproductive gland of approximately 3 - 4 cm in diameter having a mass of about 20 grams in a male between 20 and 30 years of age. In a young boy the prostate weighs between 3 and 6 grams. In the average healthy 30 year old male the prostate is about the size of a walnut; it remains about that size until about age 50 then slowly begins to increase in volume and mass, its tissues changing or differentiating with advancing age. It may weigh more than 50 grams in a fifty to sixty year old male. Some men have prostate glands that may grow more rapidly than others, often leading to rapid growth of benign tissue and in some cases triggering the development of malignancy or cancer; the benign growth of tissue, however, does not promote the development of prostate cancer. There is no single known reason for any change in the condition of a man's prostate gland, its progressive enlargement with age or in the development of malignancy.

The prostate gland is normally underdeveloped before puberty and slowly increases in size when testosterone levels increase during puberty. The **adrenal glands** located at the anterior or top end of each kidney also produce small amounts of male and female androgens (hormones) before puberty and continue to produce androgens such as androstenedione, a form of testosterone, well beyond puberty. About 95 percent of the testosterone in males after puberty is produced by the testes and continues to be produced throughout life. Testosterone is secreted into the blood to other parts of the body including the skeletal muscles as well as into the prostate gland. Testosterone, as mentioned earlier, is converted into dihydrotestosterone for the normal functioning of the prostate gland.

The prostate gland is located at the base of the bladder just above the lower rectum. This gland actually surrounds the **urethra** which is about 20 cm in total length below the neck of the bladder and continues to the penis; the small portion that passes through the prostate is called the prostatic urethra and the membranous urethra is located between the prostate and the penis. The base of the prostate is wider than the apex that sits just below the bladder. The main function of the urethra is to transport urine from the bladder and the reproductive semi-fluid substances containing sperm cells known as semen; the urethra courses its way through to the penis. Semen is a mixture of sperm cells made in the testes and consists of the fluids that the prostate and the seminal vesicles produce that are secreted during a man's ejaculation.

The prostate gland consists of three general histological and distinctive glandular zones. The peripheral zone consists of 70 – 75 percent of glandular tissue and is just inside the capsule which is like the outer skin of a plum. It is located closest to the rectum and is easily felt during a rectal examination and fortunately the site of the majority of prostate cancer tumours. The central zone occupies about 20 – 25 percent of glandular tissues that hold the gland together and grow as a man ages; prostate cancer is seldom found in this zone and, if it does develop, it tends to be slow growing. The transition zone occupies about 5 – 10 percent of the prostate and surrounds the urethra; it continues to grow as a man ages and is often the site of benign growth. About 20 percent of prostate cancer tumours originate in the transition zone. The anterior zone is in front of the gland and is composed mainly of smooth muscles that function in contractions during an ejaculation. The prostate is a very active gland producing and secreting a milky-looking substance consisting of nutrients as well as the prostate specific antigen (PSA) enzyme. During ejaculation, secretions from both the prostate gland and seminal vesicles are required to nourish sperm cells and keep them alive for several hours. Without prostatic secretion, sperm cells would lack the necessary nutrients for their metabolism and the ability to swim, both factors that can result in male sterility.

The histology or tissue arrangement of the prostate consists of many saccular glands and ducts or tiny tubes; other tissues that are associated with the prostate gland include important nerves and blood vessels. Nerves that innervate the prostate gland are necessary to empty its contents during an ejaculation. The **neurovascular bundles** necessary for erectile potency run alongside the prostate. The **cavernous nerves** specifically run posterolateral to the prostate and do not pass directly on its lateral surface. The discharge of semen from the erect penis at the moment of the sexual climax is known as ejaculation and controlled by tiny nerves on the prostate gland. Blood vessels are used to transport testosterone and nutrients to the prostate; substances such as glycoproteins may leave the prostate and pass into the bloodstream. Cancer cells and proteins may also pass out of the diseased prostate gland into the lymphatic system, and specifically enter into the lymph nodes. I will discuss the importance of the glycoprotein, referred to as the **prostate specific antigen** or **PSA**, and metastasis or spreading of cancer in subsequent chapters.

Generalized Function of the Reproductive System

As a man ages his prostate gland progressively enlarges and is mainly under the influence of the male sex hormones, testosterone and dihydrotestosterone. The glycoprotein enzyme or prostate specific antigen, is made in the epithelial cells of the prostate that is used as a marker in the early detection of prostate problems including prostate cancer. As a man ages his PSA value generally increases; any changes in prostate enlargement, benign or cancerous growth, will elevate the PSA values. Cancer cells and tumours produce more PSA than non-cancerous tissue. Thus the PSA is a good marker for the presence of prostate cancer. Since protein synthesis is directed by **deoxyribonucleic acid** (DNA) or genes, it appears that changes on the genes would promote more PSA synthesis than normal. The tiny nerve fibres running alongside the prostate are necessary for erectile potency and run directly to the penis. Restoring potency and erectile dysfunction are discussed in Chapter 8. The nerves in the prostate gland itself are involved with the secretion of prostatic fluids during ejaculation. A noted Dutch urologist, Pieter Donker, first identified the carvernous nerves in a deceased male. Drs. Donker and Walsh discussed the importance of those nerves and specific location; urologist Walsh later perfected the nerve-sparing operation during surgical removal of the prostate gland. The prostate gland, incidentally, has nothing to do with a man's ability to have an erection. Erection is mainly due to the action of the neurovascular bundles consisting of nerves, blood vessels and the accompanying physiological activity on the penis. If the prostate is removed by surgery or **radical prostatectomy** it does not follow that the person will become sexually impotent and cannot experience ejaculation; impotence or erectile dysfunction results mainly when the neurovascular bundles to the penis are severed or damaged during surgery or by radiation. The nerve-sparing technique may not be performed with every surgery procedure. The extent of the cancer on the prostate, either marginal or confined, determines whether nerve-sparing can be performed.

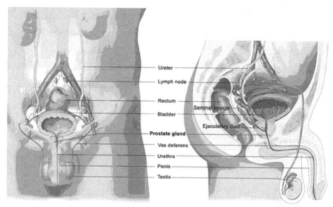

Figure 1.1: Front and Side Views of the Male Reproductive and Urinary Systems. Image adapted from the National Cancer Institute Visuals.

The secretion of prostatic fluid is a continuous process in the adult male life and it accounts for over 35 - 40 percent of seminal fluid of the ejaculate in a man's semen; the remaining ejaculate comes from fluids in the **seminal vesicles** and contributes to about 60 percent of the semen. **Spermatozoa** or sperm cells account for about 1 - 2 percent of the total ejaculate. A lesser known gland is the Cowper's, a pair of glands located posterior to the prostate that secretes a tiny amount of seminal fluid consisting of antibacterial and alkaline substances – it is the pre-ejaculatory fluid since any microbes and acidity should be removed from the urethra prior to ejaculation. Alkaline substances in semen counteract any acidity in the vagina so as to allow sperm cells to remain active. Sperm cells are continuously being produced in the **testes** and are temporarily stored in the **epididymis,** a long convoluted tube located on the lower side of the testis and when uncoiled could reach a length of over four metres. Maturation of sperm cells is carried out in the epididymis in order to enhance male fertility. After maturing for several days, sperm cells then pass from the epididymis into the **vas or ductus deferens** on the way to the urethra. The **ejaculatory** ducts are connected to both the seminal vesicles and prostate gland that secrete the seminal fluids into the urethra during a man's ejaculation.

When the prostate is removed, a man becomes sterile but he may not necessarily become impotent. Some time after surgery, a man may still continue to have sexual intercourse and experience an ejaculation but without the seminal fluids present in his ejaculate. After radical prostatectomy for prostate cancer a man will, therefore, have a dry ejaculate – no semen being present as both the prostate gland and seminal vesicles are surgically removed. Erectile dysfunction or impotence is naturally an important concern with most men before and after treatment for prostate cancer. The pioneer of the nerve-sparing technique, Dr. Patrick Walsh of Johns Hopkins University, reported that erectile potency can be preserved even when one neurovascular bundle is sacrificed. Walsh performed his first nerve-sparing prostatectomy in 1982 on a 52 year old man who regained his sexual potency one year later. Most urologists today will perform the nerve-sparing technique when surgery is required; patients need to be warned, however, that the latter procedure may not be possible with every radical prostatectomy or surgery procedure. Radical prostatectomy, nerve-sparing technique and its limitations are discussed in Chapter 7.

If a man suffers from erectile dysfunction after surgery or following radiation, the physician may suggest several options to the patient for achieving an erection. Please refer to Chapter 8 for details of treatment options available to men who become sexually impotent. A patient after consultation with his urologist and spouse or partner, may decide upon a particular treatment option for his erectile dysfunction. The efficacy of drugs such as Viagra, Cialis and Levitra has been tested for improving potency and are now widely available by prescription. In Chapter 8, a number of controlled experiments have been cited with these modern drugs. Prostate Centres, Cancer Agency Libraries, offices of urologists, the Canadian Male Sexual Health Council, provide literature and audiovisual materials to inform men about erectile dysfunction after treatment for prostate cancer. There are websites too that provide information on sexual dysfunction for patients. Three recommended websites are: www.malehealth.com, www.cmshc.org, and www.impotence.org. A list of useful websites on prostate cancer and health information is provided at the end of this book.

Hormonal Interactions

The biology of the prostate and treatment options will not be complete without an understanding of the role of the endocrine glands that produce hormones. Hormones are substances that are produced and secreted by specific glands in our body and transported elsewhere to cause physiological changes. For example, the pancreas produces insulin that is transported to many organs and tissues for sugar metabolism. The pituitary gland is about one centimetre in diameter, located in the mid-ventral side of the brain and is known as the master gland because it produces and secretes many hormones. The interactions of hormones that are produced in the brain, testes and adrenal gland located just above the kidney, can be complex but need to be understood in order to appreciate how androgen deprivation therapy works. Hormones are secreted into the blood from one part of the body and mainly from endocrine glands such as the pituitary to cause an effect on another part or organ of the body. Indeed, hormonal therapy for prostate cancer applies the principles of feedback relationships of hormones produced by the testes and related endocrine glands, such as the pituitary and hypothalamus. The hypothalamus is situated in the region just above the pituitary gland.

Several glands throughout the body target, either directly or indirectly, the activity of the prostate gland. These endocrine glands that affect the prostate are the testes, hypothalamus, pituitary and to a lesser extent, the adrenal glands. Specialized cells of the testis known as Leydig cells or interstitial cells (located outside the tiny tubule of cells) secrete testosterone, the male sex hormone, which is essential for the metabolism of prostatic cells. Testosterone is responsible for establishing the male sex characteristics such as body hair growth, skeletal growth, increase in musculature, supporting development of sperm cells, a man's libido (sex drive), and voice changes after puberty. In addition to producing the hormone testosterone, the testes consist of many microscopic tubules or seminiferous tubules. Surrounding each tubule are cells that divide to reduce the number of chromosomes of the cell by one-half or 23 chromosomes per sex cell, that later differentiates into mature sperm cells by assuming tiny tails or flagellae in order to enable them to be motile and travel as far as the fallopian tubes in the female reproductive tract. From the tubules in the testes, the newly formed sperm cells travel to a holding area, the epididymis, for further development and maturation before they are able to fertilize the egg.

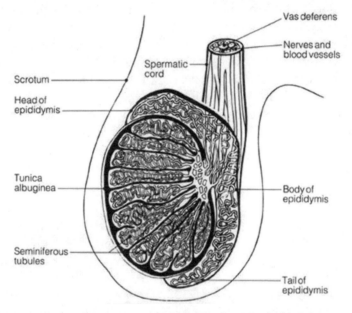

Figure 1.2: Section of the testis or testicle where sperm cells and testosterone are produced. Adapted from the National Cancer Institute Visuals.

Previously mentioned is the importance of the hypothalamus and pituitary glands and their influence on the testis. There are important feedback relationships between and among those latter three endocrine glands. The hypothalamus secretes a luteinizing hormone releasing hormone (LHRH) which stimulates the pituitary gland to secrete its own hormones. The pituitary hormones are stimulated by LHRH from the hypothalamus to allow for the secretion of luteinizing hormone (LH). LH is secreted into the blood, like all hormones, and targets the Leydig cells of the testes to produce testosterone. The pituitary gland produces many hormones and one in particular is a **follicle stimulating hormone** or FSH that is necessary for the production of sperm cells. The information presented on hormones can be somewhat confusing but Chapter 9 discusses the importance of anti-androgens such as LHRH analogs as an important form of therapy for treating patients with prostate cancer.

To briefly summarize, LHRH from the hypothalamus stimulates the production of LH in the pituitary gland; the latter hormone targets and stimulates the interstitial or Leydig cells of the testis that are responsible for the production of the male sex hormone, testosterone. FSH, on the other hand, targets the seminiferous tubule cells of the testis for the production of sex cells before they enter the long coiled tube or epididymis. FSH teams up with LH to prompt the testis to produce testosterone. Both LH and FSH from the pituitary gland are part of normal sexual development including a man's ability to make sperm cells. Without the hypothalamus or pituitary, the testes could not perform their role as sex organs; that is, in the production of sperm cells and the secretion of testosterone. Testosterone from the testes and a small amount of male androgens from the adrenals both activate the prostate gland; the adrenals too are under the influence of the pituitary gland.

Some investigators suspect that as a man ages his prostate becomes more sensitive to testosterone even though there is less of it, starting at an age of 40 years. Interestingly, a man's level of estrogen, the female sex hormone, (and men have small amounts of it), remains fairly constant and may even slightly increase as he ages; researchers speculate that even with that small amount of estrogen and the lowering of testosterone, it would trigger benign growth of the prostate. Some scientists also speculate that the imbalance of estrogen and testosterone may also trigger malignancy of the prostate but more research is needed to confirm this hypothesis. **Adrenocorticotropic hormone,** or ACTH, from the pituitary gland stimulates the adrenal cortex to secrete androstenedione, a male androgen; the latter hormone functions like testosterone and targets the prostate cells in much the same way like testosterone. As mentioned earlier, the enzyme 5-alpha reductase converts testosterone into the prostatic hormone, dihydrotestosterone (DHT). DHT triggers the synthesis of certain growth factors in the nucleus of the prostate cell which is known to cause benign growth and promote prostate cancer. When a man is taking hormone therapy for controlling his cancer, testosterone levels drop and DHT is blocked that would inhibit the growth factors and suppress or control cancer or benign cell growth.

The growth of tumours, either benign or malignant, with the tendency to grow and divide, is stimulated by the action of testosterone, dihydrotestosterone and certain growth factors. The precise way tumours develop is still to be determined but changes in the genes or affected DNA molecule start the process of abnormal development. If the prostate gland is denied its major ingredient, that is testosterone, then cancer or any abnormal development may be eliminated or suppressed. It is well known that in some men, especially among eunuchs who possess very low levels of testosterone, or in men who had their testicles removed prematurely due to testicular cancer or other disease, prostate cancer never develops. Castration or orchiectomy as a form of androgen deprivation therapy will be discussed later as one way to control advanced prostate cancer. When the levels of testosterone drop, the metabolic activity of the prostate gland will be restricted and cancer activity will be suppressed. Figure 1.3 below illustrates some of the hormonal interactions discussed above.

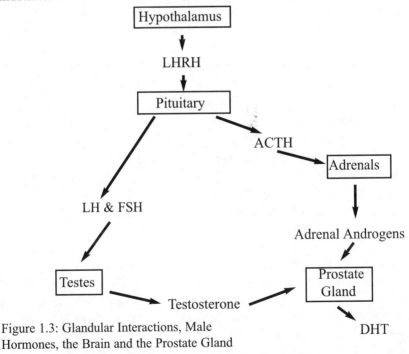

Figure 1.3: Glandular Interactions, Male Hormones, the Brain and the Prostate Gland

Genetic Markers

Genetic markers are also being investigated in many cancer cases. Patient history is being investigated for genetic lines of cancer and other diseases. Each cell, with a few exceptions, has a nucleus that contains tiny rod-like bodies known as **chromosomes.** In each chromosome there are hundreds or thousands of **genes** depending on the chromosome size; genes are segments of the universal chemical and found in tiny organisms such as viruses and bacteria, in all plants, animals and in humans. That universal biochemical molecule is **deoxyribonucleic acid or DNA** for short. The DNA is a double helical twisted molecule that was discovered by Drs. James Watson and Francis Crick in early 1950s; it is long when it is unwound and has profound significance to the survival and evolution of the species. DNA provides the information necessary to synthesize proteins and enzymes; exact copies of DNA will pass from one generation of cells to the next during cell division process. Most people have heard of DNA testing to determine an individual's description in criminal cases – each person has a specific DNA and identical twins have exact copies. Similarities of DNA or genes are also found when determining ancestral lines. The DNA is able to change or mutate and these changes may lead to genetic disorders and cancers. In the next chapter a basic understanding on how some cancers develop due to changes in the DNA will be discussed.

Genetic markers in brothers and fathers with prostate cancer are being investigated for genetic linkages and some of them have been discovered. The Genome Project has mapped the tens of thousands of genes, and many research laboratories have discovered genes which predispose some men to having prostate cancer. Several prostate cancer susceptibility genes were identified on chromosome numbers 1, 4, 5, 7, 8, 16, 19, 20 and on the X and Y chromosomes. Many more genes for cancers will be found with the ongoing research. Not all of the data is clear with linking prostate cancer with the above mentioned chromosomes or gene sites. Humans carry 23 pairs of chromosomes per cell including the sex chromosomes XX for females and XY for males. A cancer suppressor gene was identified on chromosome 16 and shows a strong link with prostate cancer. The function of this suppressor gene is lost or disabled in prostate cancer patients. A tumour suppressor gene is one in which a loss of function contributes to the development of cancer.

A large cohort group of families affected with having prostate cancer was studied using blood samples. An abnormal form of chromosome number one (of the 23 pairs) has been identified as a carrier of a prostate cancer gene, known as a hereditary prostate cancer 1 or HPC1. The X chromosome, one of the sex chromosomes, has also been implicated in prostate cancer in families and confirmed by research in Germany by Dr. Bochum and colleagues studying 104 prostate cancer families. The X chromosome present in all males is inherited from mothers. As mentioned above, the inactivity of a tumour suppressor gene on chromosome number 16 was reported as having another strong linkage to prostate cancer. Chromosomal inheritance plays a significant part in promoting prostate cancer (and other cancers such as breast cancer) when a mutation occurs in the DNA of those affected genes. What are some of the causes of prostate cancer? As mentioned earlier, eunuchs or men who were castrated at an earlier age never get prostate cancer. Testosterone activity on the prostate, inheritance or genetics factors, and dietary considerations such as a high consumption of fats, or lack of certain minerals and vitamins collectively play important roles in advancing prostate cancer. The role of diet is discussed in Chapter 4 as important preventative considerations for prostate cancer.

Chapter 2

Cancer: An Introduction

By reading this chapter you will learn:

- How does cancer begin?
- What is the role of DNA and mutations in cancer development?
- The importance of oncogenes and tumour suppressor genes.
- How do cancer cells behave?
- What is prostate intraepithelial neoplasia or PIN?
- What happens when normal cell division is affected?
- Identifying prostate cancer genes, p53 and PCA3 gene, and a new prostate cancer marker.
- Known environmental factors that promote malignancy.
- Message on prevention to reduce the risk of cancer.

How does Cancer Begin

Research has solved some of the mysteries of cancer during the last 50 years. When we speak of cancer we think of only a few specific diseases that affect the general population. There are, in fact, more than 100 different types of cancer; however, only the more common forms such as lung, breast, prostate, colon, skin, lymphoma or brain cancers are generally presented in detail since these common cancers affect the population at large. Cancer research is being conducted in many laboratories and clinics at an enormous cost and this research seems to be to be a lifelong task with new discoveries being reported every week in eminent journals. Be cautious of the many reports in daily newspapers and some magazines on cancer cures and research. Some newspapers falsely interpret scientific findings or the entire story on the research is not always reported. This chapter addresses some of the basic biology of cancer research.

How a cancer develops is still not completely understood. A cancer cell looks and behaves quite differently than a normal cell. Changes in the cell's deoxyribonucleic acid or DNA are well known to trigger abnormal cell growth. Cells of a tumour generally descend from an ancestral cell or from cells through an accumulation of genetic changes or mutations on the DNA or gene. The DNA is a long twisted double helical biochemical molecule located within each chromosome and is known to direct the synthesis of proteins and enzymes through transcribed nuclear ribonucleic acid or RNA. RNA is made, or transcribed, from the DNA or genes and is involved principally in protein synthesis. Proteins processed in the cytoplasm through our genes using RNA molecules help with cell metabolism and general bodily function. The process of protein synthesis goes on around the clock or we would not be able to survive as a species; all organisms, including viruses and bacteria, synthesize proteins. Some proteins become functional enzymes through cell processing and are used in biochemical reactions. For example, there are enzymes in our digestive tract that help to convert the foods we eat into useable smaller molecules such as sugars that are absorbed from the intestine. The presence of abnormal proteins or enzymes or the absence of some of them may often signal the presence of faulty genes in our body. A faulty gene refers to a mutation or change on the DNA. The DNA molecule is tightly wrapped inside the chromosome and each chromosome is different than others in its size and genetic composition. Each chromosome has a definite number of genes and may number in the hundreds or thousands depending on the chromosome size. Individuals inherit half their chromosomes from each parent, the egg having 22 plus the X chromosome, and the sperm carrying 22 plus the X or Y chromosome. The X chromosome carries many more genes than the Y chromosome and the XX combination at the time of fertilization will develop into a female while the XY combination will become a male offspring; there are a few exceptions to this combination in the human population.

The work that was completed and still ongoing with the Genome Project has identified many genetic disorders and mapped thousands of genes. Celera Genomics, headed by Dr. Craig Venter, announced in 2000 that it had sequenced and assembled the entire human genome. The mapping of genes by scientists has been ongoing well before Venter's announcement and the search for the proteins and enzymes of specific genes will continue for many more years. In November of 1996, as reported in the journal of Science, genetic linkages for prostate cancer were identified on the long arm of chromosome number one. Two breast cancer genes were identified in 1994 and 1995. The investigation on gene mapping and knowing what each gene is responsible for will take many more years to unravel. The identified prostate gene is named Hereditary Prostate Cancer 1or HPC 1 and when mutated, is believed to be associated with familial prostate cancers. A gene on the X chromosome, inherited in males from mothers, has also been implicated in promoting hereditary prostate cancer. As mentioned in the last chapter, other chromosomes identified as carrying prostate cancer genes are located on numbers 1, 4, 5,7, 8, 16, 19, 20 and the X and Y chromosomes. The numbering of pairs of chromosomes using special staining techniques, by the arranging them according to size from 1 to 22 and XX or XY, and displaying them from photographs is known as a **karyotype.** The karyotype procedure is also useful in genetic studies and in identifying certain abnormalities. Modern methods are now being used to sequence the genes, to identify abnormalities, and to develop new drugs that would target cancer cells and genetic disorders.

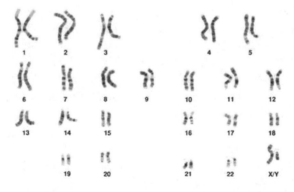

Figure 2.1: Normal Male Karyotype of 22 pairs of autosomes and one pair of sex chromosomes. Adapted from the National Cancer Institute Visuals.

Three prostate cancer susceptibility genes have been reported by Dr. Xu and colleagues at the Center for Human Genomics in North Carolina and were linked to different regions of chromosome number 1 by studying 159 hereditary prostate cancer families. At the Marshfield Medical Research Foundation in Wisconsin, Dr. Zhang and investigators demonstrated that regions of chromosomes 1, 4, 5, 7, 8, 16 and 19 might carry genes that predispose men to prostate cancer. At the Mayo Clinic in Rochester, Dr. Slager and colleagues provided strong evidence to show that chromosome 19 harbours a gene for prostate tumour aggressiveness. At the University of Maryland School of Medicine, Dr. Zheng and collaborators reported a region on chromosome number 20 with having a link to a prostate cancer susceptibility gene by studying the 159 hereditary prostate cancer families cited above. Human prostate cancer is linked to the X chromosome and this connection was confirmed in 104 German prostate cancer families studied by Dr. Bochum and colleagues. The hypothesis that deletion of the Y chromosome-specific genes is associated with prostate cancer was published by Dr. Perinchery at Veterans Affairs Medical Center in San Francisco – the loss of Y-chromosome-specific genes may suggest a role in pathogenesis of prostate cancer disease. More research is needed to confirm prostate cancer gene sites and what metabolites, if any, are affected by those genes.

Two general categories of genes are involved in the promotion of cancer when there is a mutation. The *proto-oncogenes* are known to stimulate cell division and promote normal cell growth. When proto-oncogenes are mutated they become cancer genes or *oncogenes;* the latter genes cause cells to become overactive, resulting in rapid and abnormal cell division when cancer causing agents affect the cell's DNA. The activated oncogenes would promote cancer cell growth. The normal cell cycle then goes out of balance through genetic mutations and normal cell division process or mitosis gets out of control. Cancer cells also divide and even grow more rapidly than normal cells, becoming quite independent by being nourished by newly formed blood vessels. A second kind of gene, known as a *tumour suppressor* gene, normally places checks and balances on the cell growth or cell division in the presence of specific proteins. When a tumour suppressor gene becomes mutated, those controlling proteins for normal cell division are inactivated and the process of cell division becomes unchecked. A tumour suppressor gene for prostate cancer was reported by an Emory University scientist and is believed to be carried on chromosome number 16. The latter tumour suppressor gene is "a transcription factor that functions to regulate the expression of other genes." That gene on chromosome 16 was also identified as having a strong linkage to prostate cancer.

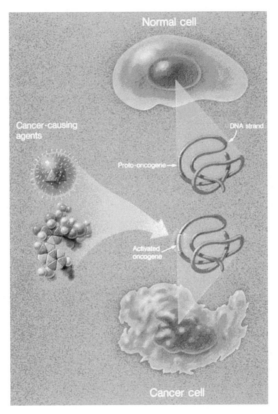

Figure 2.2: Oncogene activation. Adapted from the National Cancer Institute Visuals

Mutations begin within a cell when a gene or genes change by alterations of the DNA or through an accumulation of environmental factors such as cigarette smoke or solar radiation. The result of genetic mutations within the DNA or genes may lead to the development of tumours or cancer. Radiation for treatment of cancer is designed to alter genes and kill specific cancer cells. When mutations occur on the affected genes, cells then increase their ability to proliferate or reproduce when they should behave normally. Those abnormal or mutated cells divide rapidly and promote tissue growth, resulting in the condition known as hyperplasia. The latter term should not be confused with prostate hyperplasia. Tumour development occurs in stages and any new growth may be either benign or cancerous. When clinicians observe cancer cells they recognize significant differences in the cell's shape, size and nuclear composition as compared with normal cells. The nucleus of a cancerous cell is unusually large and the shape of the cell is generally altered and deformed. Prostate cancer cells therefore generally vary in shape and size from the normally well differentiated cells when clinicians observe tissues under the microscope after a biopsy. Cell differentiation and grading of prostate cancer cells will be discussed in Chapter 6.

Prostate cancer cells begin to grow into microscopic pre-cancerous tumours that are not palpable or cannot be felt by the attending physician during a digital rectal examination. Cells may remain confined to that tissue then later differentiate and may grow into a lump or swelling. It may take many years before any pre-cancerous cells become life threatening. Many men over the age of 60 years carry pre-cancerous prostate cells that pose no immediate risk. Prostate intraepithelial neoplasia or PIN refers to cells that surround the ducts of the gland and are comparable to carcinoma cells that are not life threatening. High grade PIN is equivalent to pre-cancerous cells that may be a warning sign much like a rise in the PSA level. PIN is discovered by biopsy after a suspicious PSA value is found. It is recommended that men who have high grade PIN and an elevated PSA should have a repeat biopsy three to four months later. Cancer cells can only be detected under a microscope and are not palpable or cannot be felt by rectal examination unless cells develop into a lumpy mass of tissue - the doctor can then feel a lump if cancer is present in a man's prostate through the digital rectal examination. The peripheral zone of the prostate is the common site of adenocarcinomas or palpable cancerous growths. Biopsy of tissue is meant to detect cancerous cells even if a palpable tumour is not identified in an early staging of prostate cancer. A lump, if cancerous, may originate or stay at that site for an indefinite period of time. Changes may continue to occur in cancer cells at a localized site that could later differentiate and become more aggressive in nature; such cancer cells may pass into the blood or lymph system. The spreading of cancer cells onto adjacent or distant tissues is known as metastasis. Prostate cancer cells may escape the capsule of the gland and enter the seminal vesicles and adjacent lymph nodes. The individual will still be unaware that his cancer is behaving aggressively and is unable to experience any symptoms of his cancer at this stage. If the tumour is less than 1 cm to 2 cm in diameter and confined to the prostate, the prognosis is excellent for a curative treatment with surgery. Details of treatment options will be discussed in subsequent chapters based on the results of diagnostic tests. Distant metastases of prostate cancer may appear in the bones when the cancer has advanced. Treatment options for advanced prostate cancer are available throughout Canada and medical care would control its progression, reduce symptoms as well as improve the quality of a man's life.

The Cell's Clock

Cell division is a continuous process in most tissues and organs; some tissues carry out mitosis or cell division more frequently than others. Red blood cells, for example, are completely replaced about every four months - the red bone marrow continually undergoes cell division. The cells lining the intestine regenerate every few days. Skin cells are replaced every day with new cells when the older ones slough off. The simplified cell cycle below explains the cyclical phases and identifies where abnormal activities may occur. Cell division is an ongoing process with very few mistakes being made by nature. But mistakes do occur within human cells. In general, a normal cell grows and uses the nutrients that enter it for its metabolism. DNA and RNA work in unison to produce proteins and enzymes well before the cell begins to divide. Organelles such as the mitochondria are present in plant and animal cells to generate cellular energy in order for the cell to function and to maintain the life of the organism. During most of the cell cycle, the cell is synthesizing substances, using nutrients, growing, producing and using energy for its survival and getting ready for its division. During a short time span of the cell cycle, the cell division process occurs when chromosomes divide into equal numbers and the cell membrane then finally divides forming two exact copies of the mother cell. Specific "signals" or proteins are actively functional in promoting or restraining cell growth well before the DNA of a cell begins to replicate or divide. The normal cell cycle appears to be deranged when DNA (or a gene) becomes mutated. Specific proteins that run the signals or switches for the "on" or "off" steps for a normal cell division process could go missing or there may be too many of them being produced, thus interfering with the normal division process. When a mutation occurs in the DNA, protein synthesis and the normal cell division process become deranged.

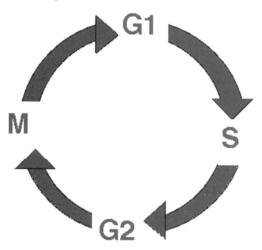

Figure 2.3: The Generalized Cell Cycle

A cell normally enlarges in the gap 1 phase (G1) of the above cell cycle before DNA replicates in S phase or synthesis stage. The G1 phase is known as the period of cell activity and growth before the actual replication of DNA in the S phase could begin. If a mutation occurs during the G1 phase, at that specific site of the cell cycle, the normal duplication of DNA may not be occur; sometimes repair is possible to ward off any mutations. The normal protein switches that operate for the progression of the cell cycle are turned off when a cell is mutated, leading to an abnormal cell division. That mutated cell is likely to become cancerous in the course of its development. Such a cell will continue to divide in its own way, resulting in the development of a tumour. Abnormal prostate cancer cells can become either benign or malignant. Researchers have identified certain protein "signals" known as *cyclins* that increase or decrease in amounts as the cell cycle unfolds. Normal cyclin levels are needed for the cell to proceed from the G1 phase to complete cell division or mitosis at the M stage above. An increasing level of G1-cyclins bind to their cyclin-dependent kinases (cdk) and signal the cell to prepare the chromosomes to divide. Breast cancer cells are known to synthesize an *over-production* of the cyclin proteins that interfere with normal cell division.

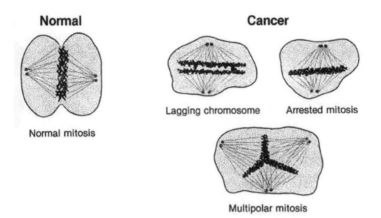

Figure 2.4: Normal and abnormal cell division or mitosis. Adapted from the National Cancer Institute Visuals.

Gene Action and Cancer

Without getting into the details of the research, a mutated cell produces an over-production of specific proteins such as cyclins that have been implicated in some human cancers. The over-production of those cyclin proteins results in an over-stimulation of the events in the cell cycle. The result is an excessive growth of cells that appear to look different than the surrounding cells. The switches that turn on and off the cell cycle also seem to exist in different forms. For example, a protein switch is produced when the p53 gene that is a small segment of the DNA molecule, indirectly expresses that specific protein within the cell's nucleus before its synthesis in the cell cytoplasm. That important protein synthesized through the p53 gene is simply known as the p53 protein. When the normal p53 protein is altered due to a mutation of the p53 gene, cancers would subsequently develop. Dr. Bert Volgelstein of the Johns Hopkins Oncology Centre first discovered that when p53 gene was damaged or mutated the body was more susceptible to cancers. Mutations in p53 are detected in more than 50 percent of all human cancers including lung, breast, bladder and brain cancers.

The p53 gene has been referred to the "guardian of the genome" and is a key player in protecting against cancer since it produces the regulatory protein p53. The p53 protein normally controls normal DNA replication and allows the cell to complete its cycle. Interactions between the p53 protein and the DNA stimulate another gene to produce a protein referred to as p21 protein. The latter protein interacts with yet another protein, cyclin-dependent kinase2, in order to stimulate cell division. The p53 protein also promotes the suicide of cells that have the tendency of becoming abnormal. The process is a biological phenomenon known as **apoptosis** or programmed cell death because the cell advances through a series of steps that brings about its destruction or by committing suicide. The p53 gene mapped on chromosome 17 may block tumour growth by inducing apoptosis and by causing reversible arrest in the G1 phase of the cell cycle. Mutations of the p53 tumour suppressor gene are generally believed to be a late event in the progression of prostate cancer; a finding reported by Dr. Downing and others in the *Canadian Journal of Urology*. In 1996, a carcinogen in cigarette smoke was first identified to cause mutations on the p53 gene. This carcinogen in cigarettes was identified as pyro[a]benzene and is the cause of one form of human lung cancer. The research finding with this chemical provides a direct link between the identified cigarette smoke carcinogen and human lung cancer. Certain environmental factors are well known to promote cancers but it is the first time that a defined carcinogen found in cigarettes was implicated as a culprit for promoting lung cancer. A large number of harmful substances and carcinogens have been identified in cigarette smoke. Once cancer appears in the lungs after a long exposure to carcinogens in cigarette smoke, the survival time for the patient is generally short. The human species, however, is able to counteract many "mistakes" that are made within the body and repair them before they become life-threatening. Antioxidants play important roles in preventing free radicals from doing harm to cells.

When geneticists examine the chromosome they can identify genetic abnormalities by using new and advanced techniques. Many genetic disorders and cancers were identified from chromosomal studies. Cervical cancer, for example, reveals abnormalities in chromosome number 8. The normal human cell consists of 22 pairs of chromosomes and one pair of sex chromosomes, XX in females and XY in males. Chromosome number 17 is known to carry breast cancer genes. Unfortunately we do not have all the answers on how the prostate cancer genes identified thus far trigger prostate cancer; more research will shed light on oncogenes, tumour suppressor genes and the proteins that regulate the cell cycle. The new technology on gene mapping will identify many more cancers and make it possible to treat diseases before they become life-threatening. Ethical concerns may arise when individuals who are identified early in life with genetic disorders or diseases such as breast cancer or any disease such as Huntington's disease. Do you want to know whether you are a carrier of the cystic fibrosis gene? How will you cope with the knowledge that a life-threatening disease could develop later in life? New therapies will also emerge with the advancing research on gene therapy, from stem cell research or through genetic engineering. A clinical trial for gene therapy for prostate cancer is being launched by Dr. Nick James and his team at the University of Birmingham in England. Tough decisions lie ahead for those individuals who take genetic tests, knowing that they may be carriers of the so-called bad genes.

Celera Genomics, the Human Genome Project, and international research laboratories are working on identifying the proteins and enzymes that are affected by mutated genes. Knowing which metabolite is missing may help in the treatment of genetic disorders and cancers. One genetic code, identified as **DD3 PCA3** or simply **PCA3,** is one of the "most prostate cancer-specific gene...and that it is a very sensitive specific marker for the detection of prostate tumor cells in a high background of normal prostate cells." Oncologist Strum stated that PCA3 is a specific gene that is profusely expressed in prostate cancer cells and is 34 times greater in malignant prostate cancer tissue than in benign prostate cancer. This result was reported in several journals including *European Urology* by Dr. DeKok and colleagues and concluded: "...multi-center studies using the validated DD3PCA3 assay can provide the first basis for the utility of molecular diagnostics in clinical urological practice." A report from a Quebec-based scientific company DiagnoCure, and discussed in Urology (Elsevier) of a new urine test that may replace the PSA. The molecular urine-base genetic test for detection of prostate cancer was reported and named **uPM3.** The gene **PCA3** is one of the most specific genes yet found to be associated with prostate cancer, as noted by the Medical Director of Bostwick Laboratories where the uPM3 tumour marker is being processed. The results seem to indicate its "usefulness in detecting prostate cancer and provide some answers to the current dilemmas of early prostate cancer detection and may be particularly useful in monitoring of men with lower PSA values and those with previously negative biopsies." The new finding has great potential in reducing the number of unnecessary biopsies according to the researchers. Bostwick Laboratories has offered uPM3 as the first urine-based and genetic test for prostate cancer. Research laboratories will identify genetic markers for many cancers and develop treatment therapies that pharmaceutical companies will actively pursue. The genetics revolution will change the way cancers are diagnosed and treated.

Factors Affecting Survival

Genetic and environmental factors play significant roles in the survival of all species. The evolution of species has been naturally selected for hundreds of millions of years with large numbers of species becoming or having become extinct. Poor diet, obesity, and tobacco use account for a significant number of deaths in any human population. Every seven minutes a Canadian dies of heart disease and stroke and one Canadian dies of prostate cancer about every two hours. Epidemiological studies indicate that the incidence and death from lung cancer, colon cancer, breast cancer and prostate cancer have collectively increased over the years but heart disease is still the number one killer in Canada. Overuse of tobacco products and an over-consumption of saturated fats including red meat are contributing factors for increased mortality. Cigarette smoking can be prevented, thus reducing the incidence of lung cancer and other diseases; a high fat diet can be controlled and would significantly reduce the incidence of prostate and breast cancers including heart disease and diabetes. Japanese men living in Hawaii and California are three times more likely to develop prostate cancer than Japanese men living in Nagasaki City. Similarly, third-generation North American Japanese women have four times the risk of developing breast cancer than indigenous Japanese women. A higher fat diet, an environmental factor in the North American population, may indeed promote some forms of cancer. Genetics play a small role in cancer development but it is not the total equation when it relates to the susceptibility of having prostate cancer.

Cancer-causing agents include certain viruses and substances found in the environment. Viruses such as the papilloma virus which are sexually transmitted can radically alter normal cervical tissue into a cancerous one. Hepatitis B virus for example is known to promote liver cancer. It seems that any long exposure to certain viruses will promote cancer cell growth. The risk of stomach cancer is increased with the presence of the *Helicobacter pylori* bacteria. Radon gas from underground is known to cause lung cancer. The list of carcinogens in the workplace is extensive and include soot, synthetic fibres like asbestos, pesticides, phenoxy herbicides (in Orange Agent), benzene, diesel exhaust, second-hand tobacco smoke, to name a few. In Southeast Asia, where some children consume salty fish, there is a higher incidence of nasopharyngeal cancer in those individuals. Reducing your fat intake, using alcohol in moderation and not smoking cigarettes or chewing tobacco products will greatly reduce cancers and heart disease. Look for ways to live a healthier lifestyle.

The human body fights reactive and unstable chemicals every day including toxic by-products such as pesticides, free radicals, radiation, and environmental pollutants are known to promote cancer. If these free radicals and agents accumulate then the body's DNA is attacked causing mutations that often trigger abnormal cell growth. Our body produces enzymes that would lock up some of these bad agents; some of our foods contain anti-oxidants that render free radicals harmless. Scientists have discovered that the enzyme known as glutathione-S- transferase eliminates free radicals. What we eat also gives us additional protection against some cancers. Chapter 4 discusses the composition of foods and diet, vitamins, minerals and other factors that are effective in suppressing prostate cancer. The incidence of prostate cancer is low among Asians who consume less animal products and more plant proteins including soy products.

The pygmy chimp, the bonobo, is a complete vegetarian and does not get prostate cancer. The golden standard for a healthy lifestyle is to lower our animal fat intake, eat more vegetables, fruits and exercise more. You do not have to begin with aerobics – brisk and regular walking is always a recommended form of exercise. You can start on a slow exercise plan and then increase what you are able to do; if you are inactive, do not go out and shovel heavy snow – you could die of a heart attack! If you golf, leave the cart behind and walk. The message here is to follow a diet like a bonobo, do not smoke cigarettes, and be physically active if possible for at least 30 minutes a day. The American Cancer Society states that "cancer is largely a preventable illness – two-thirds of cancer deaths in the U.S. can be linked to tobacco use, poor diet, obesity and lack of exercise." The Canadian Cancer Society developed a *Prevention Strategy,* approved in 2004, that concluded "at least 50% of cancer cases can be prevented through healthy living, public policies and systemic changes that protect the health of Canadians. Not smoking, avoiding second-hand smoke, eating well, exercising regularly, and practicing sun protection are some key steps in reducing one's cancer risk." In addition to the above guidelines, the Canadian Cancer Society has published "Seven Steps to Health" that can be accessed from their website.

Chapter 3
Common Prostate Diseases

By reading this chapter you will learn:

- What is prostatitis?
- Symptoms and treatment for prostatitis.
- What is benign prostatic hyperplasia (BPH)?
- Determining your BPH symptom score.
- Who gets benign growth of the prostate?
- How is BPH diagnosed?
- Drugs to treat BPH, surgery and non-invasive methods.
- An introduction to prostate cancer, its incidence, and detection.

Prostatitis

Prostatitis is often caused by a bacterial infection; it is a slow progressing disease, often with painful consequences due to an inflammation of the prostate gland. Prostatitis can generally be treated with antibiotics because of bacterial infection but long-term relief from discomfort may not result. This disease, which is not cancerous, may appear suddenly in men as early as 30 years of age for no apparent reason; prostatitis may also develop from a non-bacterial condition and it may not always be 100 percent curable but can be treatable. Males affected with prostatitis may first experience difficulty passing urine, urinary burning or irritation and rectal pain as some of the many symptoms of this disease. An urologist will provide you with more information regarding the specific treatment

43

and symptoms of this disease. **Acute prostatitis** can be more easily treated as a urinary tract infection. **Chronic prostatitis** is also associated with urinary tract infections which may persist for many years and is sometimes difficult to diagnose. Persistent bacterial prostatitis may also be due to the presence of tiny stones or calculi; the latter are harmless but commonly found in middle-aged and older men. Several large clinical trials are underway that may provide more information on diagnosis and treatment of prostatitis.

Urologist Rous believes that symptoms of the non-bacterial condition probably result from an engorgement of fluid-producing glands within the prostate itself. Prostatitis may also be caused by organisms like chlamydia, mycoplasma or by urine flowing backwards into the tiny tubes or ducts of the prostate gland. In chronic prostatitis a man may complain of his frequent urination or having some difficulty in passing urine with a burning sensation. Affected individuals may also experience pain in the urethra, the tube that delivers urine from the bladder. Prolonged pain in the genitalia, anal and pelvic regions are symptomatic of chronic prostatitis. The physician may advise the affected individual to avoid spicy foods, caffeine, alcohol and smoking which would alleviate the condition of prostatitis. Treatment includes the use of anti-inflammatory drugs and antibiotics; the patient may also get some relief of his prostatitis by having more frequent ejaculations. Taking a hot bath and drinking as much water as possible to maintain a clear urine stream are recommended. Regular exercise is also recommended but riding a bike or a horse should be avoided. The prostate is like a sponge and organisms present there can spread easily. If bacteria are present and are not eradicated for acute prostatitis it may be more difficult to cure.

How do you know that you have prostatitis? A summary of symptoms include pain in the rectal area between the anus and scrotum (the perineum), pain in the testicles, blood in the urine, the need to urinate frequently, chills, difficulty in passing urine, fever, nausea, and pain during ejaculation. A man's urine may also have a foul smell when some of these symptoms develop. Check with your doctor who will investigate your symptoms and suggest appropriate treatment. Alpha blockers like Hytrin or 5-alpha-reductase inhibitors such as finasteride can also alleviate symptoms. These drugs are a second level of medication for prostatitis used to treat enlarged prostates and to improve urine flow. Be aware that inflammation due to prostatitis would elevate a man's PSA, much higher than the benign growth of the prostate. Men may needlessly worry about a high PSA level, anticipating that it may likely be prostate cancer. A rapid and sudden rise in a man's PSA it is often due to the infection and inflammation caused by prostatitis. PSA elevation may not be due to prostate cancer and is regarded as a false positive for prostate cancer. However, a man needs to be checked by having a biopsy as cancer should not be ruled out.

Benign Prostate Hyperplasia

Another disease affecting the prostate gland is **benign prostate hyperplasia** or **hypertrophy** (BPH). It is caused by the enlargement of the prostate gland that can obstruct the urethra and consequently the flow of urine. The affected individual has difficulty passing urine and it is one of the initial symptoms of BPH. As the prostate gland enlarges from within the transition zone, it begins to compress on the urethra and slowly obstructs the normal flow of urine. *Benign growth* is non-malignant and the word "*hyperplasia*" refers to any unwanted rapid growth of tissue in the prostate gland. Men should take note that the PSA value will elevate when BPH develops but its elevation is not as rapid as with prostate cancer or prostatitis. The PSA value is elevated about ten times more rapidly with prostate cancer than with benign growth tissue. The total and free PSA tests are recommended for men with BPH conditions so as to rule out any cancer. A high percent of free PSA means that you are less likely to have prostate cancer and more likely to have a BPH condition. Please refer to Chapter 5 for the total and free PSA values associated with prostate cancer and BPH. BPH is more common in older men and the incidence increases progressively with age; you should not needlessly worry about having an enlarged prostate if inflammation is discovered through a digital rectal examination. Generally nothing should be done with a benign growth of the prostate unless a person experiences severe difficulty or frequency with passing urine or experiences lower abdominal pain.

The International Prostate Symptom Score is designed to assess a man's urinary symptoms and how severe or problematic the condition may have progressed with BPH. If you are concerned about BPH and its treatment you can access and respond to the International Prostate Symptom Score to determine the severity of BPH condition. Consult the website at www.patient.co.uk to check the level of BPH. The Prostate Centre Clinic at Princess Margaret Hospital in Toronto provides information on prostate cancer, BPH, and counseling services to patients. The website is at www.prostatecentre.ca. An extensive list of websites at the end of this book provides information on a wide variety of topics on cancer and health matters. The enlargement of the prostate may cause some fine blood vessels to rupture and blood may be visible in the urine. There is no evidence to prove that having BPH will lead to prostate cancer. However, only a small percentage of men who are diagnosed with BPH are known to have prostate cancer after a biopsy is performed. About 20 percent of prostate cancers start in the transition zone where BPH is commonly found. Prostate cancer tumours found in the transition zone that encircles the urethra tend to be less aggressive and slower to metastasize than cancers in the peripheral zone.

BPH condition is observed in about 20 percent of men in their fifties, about 60 percent in men in their sixties and in about 70 percent of men in their seventies. Indeed, it is during those years when some men first realize that they actually own a prostate gland! An urologist will advise the patient of the extent of his BPH progression and what measures to take if the condition warrants treatment. What are some of the causes BPH or benign growth? Scientists do not have all the answers for the causes of BPH growth but the level of testosterone seems to be one major cause. The cause of BPH may also involve testosterone and estrogen. As a man ages his testosterone level drops and his estrogen level, which is very low, slightly increases. Some researchers speculate that a small imbalance of those two hormones may be one cause of BPH disease. Men castrated before puberty do not develop BPH. The absence of testosterone eliminates both BPH and prostate cancer. In some men, the prostate gland does not grow to full size because of a deficiency in 5-alpha-reductase, the enzyme needed to convert testosterone into dihydrotestosterone; those men do not develop BPH conditions and, incidentally, they never become bald. The drug finasteride blocks the enzyme 5-alpha-reductase and men taking it sometimes experience re-growth of hair on their heads. Some men develop larger benign growths in their prostates than others.

Benign prostatic hyperplasia or hypertrophy increases every year after the age of about forty five years. The word to stress is benign, meaning that it is not cancerous. A man's prostate gland may be twice as large at

50 years of age than when he was 20. When a man starts to develop an enlarged prostate gland with growth originating from the transition zone, he naturally experiences frequency or difficulty in urination due to the obstruction or from the slow and progressive constriction of the prostatic urethra. Having BPH growth that compresses on the urethra, it may cause the bladder wall to thicken so as to compensate for the constriction of the prostatic urethra. Male relatives at age sixty-four and younger with enlarged prostate glands were studied and found to be four times as likely to have BPH than other men who were not closely related. There seems to be a familial link among men with BPH conditions from a few reported studies in the literature. Studies carried out at Johns Hopkins suggest that BPH and prostate cancer seem to run in families.

When the prostate tissue starts to grow inwards and outwards from the transition zone, it will naturally put pressure on the urethra that carries urine from the bladder. The urethra runs right through the prostate and it seems as though it was not the most convenient anatomical invention in the male. The pressure or squeezing on the urethra builds up over the years and men will begin to wake up more frequently during the night to pass urine. A man with BPH condition experiences moments of starting

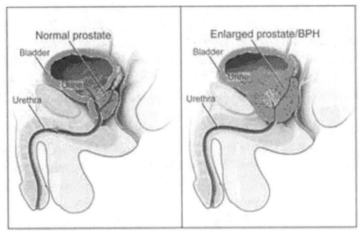

Figure 3.1 – View of the Normal and Enlarged Prostate Gland with BPH. Adapted from the National Cancer Institute Visuals

and stopping his urination and experiences the feeling of having a full bladder. You may wish to access the website on the International Prostate System Score provided in this chapter and complete the form to determine severity of your BPH symptoms. You are advised to make an appointment with an urologist if symptoms develop. An ultrasound is inserted into the rectum to determine the size of the prostate. Then a cystoscope is inserted into the penis through the urethra to determine the condition of the bladder, urethra and prostate. Other tests may be carried out to measure the pressure conditions of the bladder. The illustration in Figure 3.1 represents BPH condition compared with the normal prostate; note how the urethra is compressed and narrowed with the benign growth.

How is BPH Treated?

Before any invasive treatment for BPH begins doctors prescribe drugs to treat BPH symptoms. The well-known drug Proscar or finasteride shrinks the prostate to some degree by blocking the conversion of testosterone to its more potent analogue, **dihydrotestosterone** (DHT), which is produced in the prostate through an enzyme action with 5-alpha reductase on testosterone. Finasteride, therefore, inhibits the enzyme 5-alpha reductase so DHT production is suppressed and the benign prostate tissues begin to shrink. A double blind study with finasteride (one where the patient and the attending physician or nurse is unable to differentiate between the placebo and the real drug), was carried out by Dr. Glenn Gormley and coworkers. They found that administering 5 mg of finasteride per day to the patient was the optimum dose for treating BPH symptoms. It is interesting to note that about 50 percent of the men taking the placebo, or fake pill, in another study using finasteride reportedly felt better due in part to the psychological effect of taking the placebo. In an article in the *New England Journal of Medicine,* Dr. Paul Lange stated that finasteride or Proscar *increases testosterone level but reduces the more potent dihydrotestosterone* that is produced in the prostate gland. Dr. Catalona cautions that "because finasteride lowers serum PSA levels it could mask prostate cancer ... it may allow a worse form of cancer to emerge." Men who take Proscar should heed this warning.

If a man is taking Proscar (finasteride), Dr. Walsh recommends doubling his PSA reading in order to have a more realistic value. Medications such as Proscar and Avodart are known to reduce the PSA by about 50 percent.

A Prostate Cancer Prevention Trial, sponsored by the National Cancer Institute in the U.S., in a large study of 18 882 men over the age of 55, tested the effects of men taking 5 milligrams of finasteride daily in a placebo-controlled study. Dr. Thompson and investigators reported the findings in the *New England Journal of Medicine* and concluded, in part, that there was "an increased risk of high-grade cancer with men taking finasteride than in men in the placebo group. Sexual side effects were also more common among men in the finasteride-treated group, whereas urinary symptoms were more common in the men receiving the placebo." The results from the study also showed that finasteride prevents or delays the appearance of prostate cancer compared with the placebo group. More data is needed on finasteride research as it is thought that finasteride may alter the appearance of prostate tumours, falsely making them more aggressive, according to Dr. Alan So of the Prostate Centre in Vancouver.

Proscar, as with other drugs, has side effects including decreased libido, reduced ejaculate and sexual potency, and it may not be completely effective in increasing urinary flow; proscar is not used to treat prostate cancer. Dr. Martin Gleave at Prostate Centre at the Vancouver General Hospital reported that in "approximately one-half of patients with more established symptoms (of BPH), Proscar reduces prostate volume by 20 percent after one year of therapy and improves urinary flow rate in one-third of patients." Proscar is expensive and if it works on the patient after a one to two-year trial, it has to be taken for many years or BPH symptoms will return. Another drug used for treating BPH is Hytrin (terazosin hydrochloride) and it has shown improvement with urinary flow. There are some side-effects with Hytrin as with many other alpha blockers – be sure to ask about the side-effects and obtain any written information from the pharmacist on any medication being prescribed. Some physicians prescribe proscar and terazosin together for BPH symptoms. Another drug prescribed for treating BPH is Avodart (dutasteride) that lowers DHT to shrink the prostate gland and reduces the risk of urinary blockage. Your doctor may also prescribe other drugs that may have fewer side-effects to treat BPH. Be sure to ask about the side effects of drugs like Hytrin, Proscar or Avodart.

Ask your doctor and pharmacist which drugs to avoid when taking your prescribed medication. For example, taking alpha blockers like Hytrin and Viagra together are not recommended – the combination greatly reduces blood pressure. Some patients also take the plant derivative, saw palmetto, and patients report some success in alleviating their BPH problems. A randomized trial involving 2 939 men with symptomatic BPH were given a saw palmetto extract (*Serenoa repens*) for a mean duration of nine weeks in a placebo-controlled study including finasteride. Dr. Wilt and colleagues compared men receiving finasteride and saw palmetto and found that both groups had similar improvement in urinary tract scores. Men receiving saw palmetto had fewer adverse conditions such as erectile dysfunction. It is important to investigate the concentration of saw palmetto before using as it is an over-the-counter drug. Some products containing saw palmetto differ in their fatty acid content and not every product on the shelf at health food stores provides the same concentration. A double-blind study conducted by Dr. Bent and investigators and reported in the *New England of Medicine* on 225 men experiencing moderate to severe symptoms of BPH and using saw palmetto extract (160 milligrams twice a day), found that saw palmetto did not improve symptoms of BPH compared with the placebo group. Saw palmetto, incidentally, is not effective in preventing or treating prostate cancer.

A surgical technique used to remove benign growth is by **transurethral resection** of the prostate or TURP, is done through the urethra to alleviate the flow of urine and may need to be repeated some years later. The procedure is likened to coring an apple from the inside. The surgeon snakes a rigid or flexible lighted instrument called a **resectoscope** into the urethra while the patient is under localized anesthetic and chips away the suspicious prostate tissue as shown in Figure 3.2. Some men have referred to the latter procedure as the "roto-rooter job" commonly used by plumbers. Urologists are not too thrilled by the term. Another minor surgical method carried out infrequently is transurethral incision of the prostate or *TUIP*. The fibre optic endoscope or resectoscope makes one or two incisions in the prostate; this procedure is appropriate for patients with lesser complications of the prostate and for men with smaller prostate glands.

Several new methods are currently being investigated to treat BPH. *Laser prostatectomy* shows promise to relieve BPH symptoms with low risk of serious complications and side effects. Laser procedures have resulted in fewer transfusions, fewer strictures and requires shorter hospitalization according to the research by Hoffman and others. "Laser prosta-

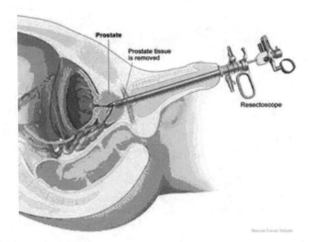

Figure 3.2: Transurethral resection procedure for BPH treatment. Adapted from the National Cancer Institute Visuals.

tectomy is as effective as TURP…in terms of safety the data suggest that the holium laser procedures are superior to TURP…" as reported by Dr. Tooher and others in *The Journal of Urology. High-Intensity Focused Ultrasound* (HIFU) heats up the prostate up to 90° Celsius for a short time. The results from HIFU are promising for BPH treatment but some patients may require re-treatment. HIFU may have a role in treating prostate cancer for men who do not want surgery as discussed in Chapter 7. Transurethral Electrovaporization of the Prostate or TUVP uses a roller-ball electrode that heats up the prostate to vaporize the tissue. Early results of this procedure for BPH also look promising. *Transurethral Microwave Thermoablation* treatment directs temperatures as high as 80° Celsius within the prostate. Dr.Larson reported that the microwave thermoablation system fulfilled the requirements for an effective and safe way to treat BPH without endangering vulnerable adjacent tissues. Dr. De la Rosette, in *The Journal of Urology* concluded: "Numerous studies unequivocally support the efficacy and safety of transurethral microwave thermotherapy for treatment of symptomatic BPH."

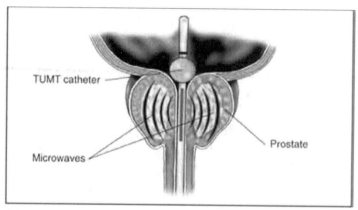

Figure 3.3: Using microwaves to treat BPH. Adapted from the National Kidney and Urologic Diseases Clearinghouse, National Institute of Health.

Prostate Cancer

The third and most serious disease of the prostate is cancer or malignancy. Prostatic cancer is the most commonly diagnosed internal cancer in men and is normally referred to as a **carcinoma** or an **adenocarcinoma.** "Adeno" means gland and "carcinoma" refers to firm or palpable tumours that generally develop in the epithelial tissues of the prostate lobes. Cancer is a disordered and abnormal growth of cells with the potential to spread or metastasize. Pre-cancerous cells that are contained within the ducts and individual glands of the prostate pose no imminent threat; these cells are referred to as *prostatic intraepithelial neoplasia* or PIN. With high grade PIN it does not mean that cancer is present but in a few years many of those cells could develop into malignant cells. In Canada, an estimated 20 500 new cases of prostate cancer was diagnosed in 2005, an increase of about 4 500 cases since the year 2000; about 4 300 deaths were estimated in 2005 for cancer cases diagnosed from previous years. The good news is that the mortality rate for prostate cancer has been significantly declining over the past ten years in Canada. In fact, the death rate from prostate cancer has dropped by 25 percent in the past ten years; a similar decline was also noted in the United States. In one province in Canada, in 2005, an estimated 3 200 new cases of prostate cancer were diagnosed in British Columbia (B.C.), the *highest rate of incidence* reported in Canada. The increasing rate of incidence of prostate cancer in B.C.

may be due to a variety of reasons. Those reasons are many and may include earlier detection with the DRE and PSA, an increase in the population of men of retirement age coming to B.C., an aging population, and many more men are becoming concerned about their health by visiting their doctors and having physical examinations. Many men are educating themselves about this disease. General practitioners are also offering the PSA test to patients who request the procedure. An Ipsos-Reid poll conducted in British Columbia found that 50 percent of men aged 45 to 75 years have had a PSA test done in the past five years.

There are no symptoms for early prostate cancer and most men are unaware of the condition. Furthermore, many cancers are microscopic, are not life-threatening or indolent in the general population, and may not be discovered until a biopsy is performed. The increase in the number of cases of prostate cancer from the 1990s to the present is probably due to earlier detection of the disease with tests such as the PSA, with more regular DRE being done by physicians as well as having a biopsy when suspicious conditions are indicated. It is also true that more men are requesting rectal exams, thus many more cases of prostate cancers are being detected earlier. The PSA test is still a very good marker for evaluation of any prostate condition; it should not be construed that the PSA by itself will determine with any certainty that a man may or may not have prostate cancer. Generally, the PSA level rises with BPH or prostatitis as well as with prostate cancer but the PSA value is elevated much higher for prostate cancer, gram for gram of tissue, than for BPH. The importance of the total and free PSA, its velocity and doubling time, PSA threshold levels and recommendations for a biopsy are discussed in Chapter 5.

Cancer cells look and behave quite differently than all other cells. Most cells multiply by cell division. A few cells in the body do not divide at all while others receive signals that allow them to divide by mitosis. The cells lining the digestive system and skin cells, for example, divide rapidly and are replaced over a short period of time. Cells also differentiate or change to take on special roles. Liver cells, for example, function differently than prostate cells and produce their own specific proteins and enzymes. Cancer cells divide rapidly, subsequently forming tumours and may continue to grow in uncontrolled ways. Some cancer cells have receptor proteins that make them effective in growing on normal tissues and organs. One type of cancer cell may grow rapidly while another type may differentiate and grow more slowly. Prostate cancer cells are generally slow growing but exceptions do occur; the word "slow" may be taken to mean years. Early prostate cancer may take from two to four years to double in size. Within the prostate gland, even when the total PSA value is low, cancer cells are known to behave aggressively. Prostate cells move from what is normal in shape to that of being disorganized and distorted. The grading of cancer cells and Gleason scores will be discussed in Chapter 6 as an important diagnostic tool to determine how aggressive a cancer is behaving or progressing.

The posterior lobe and peripheral zone of the prostate seem to be the most common sites for early cancer development and about 90 percent of aggressive cancers originate there. The transition zone is the site of about 20 percent of early prostate cancer and those tumours tend to be less aggressive. A large number of prostate cancer tumours are found in several locations of the gland or are said to be multifocal; most prostate cancers therefore are not confined to only one specific site. Thus, there is the need to remove the entire prostate gland and seminal vesicles during surgery or to radiate the entire gland for optimum treatment when cancers are multifocal. Tumour growth of the prostate may eventually leave its capsule and invade the margins and adjacent tissues. The cancer cells later spread into the blood stream and travel to the seminal vesicles and lymph nodes located adjacent to the prostate gland. Cancer cells may continue to spread or metastasize in the lymphatic system (Figure 3.4) and blood circulation, eventually to find a home in the bones.

Researchers believe that prostate cancer cells possess receptors that adhere to the surface of bone cells that allow them to continue to divide and metastasize. Cancer cells do not seem to die and serve no useful purpose. In fact, cancer cells divide more rapidly and live longer than normal cells; when cancer cells find a tissue to grow on, they can settle down, nourished by new blood vessels that develop, and continue to divide and proliferate into surrounding tissues. Subsequent chapters discuss the staging of prostate cancer, detection and diagnosis, its prevention, inheritance factors, treatment and responses to treatment.

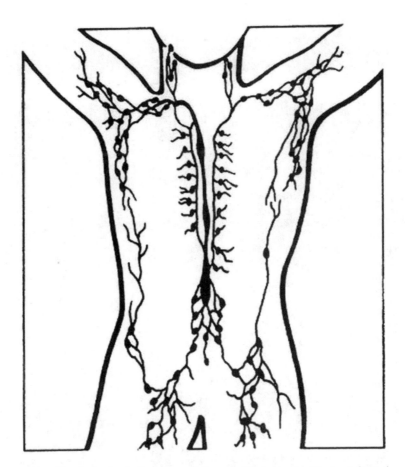

Figure 3.4 – The Lymphatic System and Lymph Nodes in the Body. Adapted from the National Cancer Institute Visuals.

Chapter 4

Prostate Cancer Data and Preventative Considerations

By reading this chapter you will learn:

- Incidence of prostate cancer, mortality rates and earlier detection.

- Preventing cardiovascular disease is a priority.

- The importance of diet in prostate cancer prevention.

- Familial/genetic linkage as a factor in developing prostate cancer.

- Is there an ethnic propensity for having prostate cancer?

- When Asians move to North America and incidence of prostate cancer.

- What do researchers say about vitamin D, ultraviolet light, a vasectomy, smoking, red wine, zinc and serum insulin growth factor?

Incidence and Mortality

Gathering information from controlled scientific studies is one way to analyze data and make more intelligent decisions about a problem. Research on prostate cancer is ongoing in many countries, especially in the United States, Canada and Europe. The public or taxpayer benefits from the research on all health matters including the testing and efficacy of new drugs as well as ways to prevent or diagnose diseases before they become too late to treat. It is not important to overburden you with figures and data presented in this chapter but you may find them useful in under-standing the progress being made on prostate cancer research, including its detection and diagnosis in Canada. One in seven Canadian men will develop clinically significant prostate cancer in his lifetime, mostly after age 70; prostate cancer is the second leading cause of cancer mortality among men, after lung cancer. More young men are being diagnosed with prostate cancer due to screening with the PSA and DRE. One out of six American men will develop prostate cancer. "Men in the U.S. have a 17.3% lifetime risk of being diagnosed with prostate cancer while the life time risk of prostate cancer deaths is 3%" according to urologist Thompson. Men of African descent in Canada and the U.S. are at a high-er risk of developing prostate cancer than those of European descent. The average age of men when diagnosed with prostate cancer in the U.S. is 69 years, at a stage in life when most men have retired or are contemplating retirement.

The incidence rate of prostate cancer cases in Canada since 1974 has doubled. The good news is that there is a significant decline in mortality rate of prostate cancer for the age group that ranges from 50 - 75 years in the Canadian population. A higher mortality rate still exists for men over 75 years of age and it is partly attributed to the late detection of their can-cer, at a stage when it is too late for any curative treatment. The relative decline in mortality rate during the past six to ten years is due to earlier detection of a man's cancer and early effective treatment. In fact, the mor-tality rates have declined by about 25 percent for prostate cancer during the past decade. However, the percentage in age-adjusted mortality rate has declined only slightly in the past ten years. In one statistic, the B.C. Cancer Agency reported that "up to 40 percent of men over 70 years of age had localized prostate cancer" when autopsies were conducted to determine the cause of death. On average, 394 Canadian men will be diag-nosed with prostate cancer every week. Autopsies conducted identified about 30 percent of men over the age of 50 years as having pre-cancerous cells in their prostate; most of those cancers were too microscopic to be considered serious or life-threatening. Urologist Scardino reported that "forty two percent of men in their seventies have some tiny clusters of cancer cells in their prostates, though the vast majority will never be dis-covered, much less cause any problems or harm." If a man is diagnosed with prostate cancer in his lifetime there is a greater than 75 percent chance that he will die of *other* causes such as heart disease, diabetes or stroke; he will most likely die with prostate cancer and not from it. In fact, men and women have more than ten times greater risk of dying of heart disease than from prostate or breast cancer in the U.S. and Canada.

The Canadian Cancer Society (CCS) publishes a booklet on cancer statistics every year so if you are interested in more information on cancers in Canada you can request a copy from their office. Check the CCS website to obtain other useful materials and information on cancer including statistics. The booklet includes the incidence, mortality, geographical patterns, graphs and tables of types of cancer for both men and women. In Canada during 2005, an estimated 76 200 men were diagnosed with cancer of all forms, and about 72 800 cancer cases were diagnosed in women. About 21 600 women were diagnosed in 2005 with breast cancer and about 5 300 died as a result. For prostate cancer, about 20 500 of men were diagnosed in 2005 and about 4 300 died from it; deaths, of course, are from cases diagnosed in past years and not necessarily from cases diagnosed in 2005. In the U.S., in 2005, there were about 232 000 new cases of prostate cancer diagnosed and about 30 500 men died from the disease.

In Canada, prostate cancer accounts for about 27 percent of all cancers diagnosed among men while the incidence of breast cancer is about 30 percent of all cancers diagnosed among women. For prostate cancer, 88 percent of new cancer cases are diagnosed in men age 60 and older. Lung cancer cases diagnosed total 16 percent of all cases of cancer among men and 14 percent for women. The mortality rate for lung cancers is still significantly higher than that of both prostate and breast cancers. In 1997, deaths from lung cancer accounted for about 32 percent of all cancer deaths in men and were reduced slightly to an estimated 29 percent in 2005. In 1997, the deaths from lung cancer in women amounted to 22 percent but had increased to an estimated 25 percent by 2005 of all cancer deaths in Canada. In 1993, lung cancer deaths in women first exceeded deaths caused by breast cancer. Among women in Canada, the mortality rate for lung cancer continues to climb steadily. In 2005, an estimated 22 200 Canadians were diagnosed with lung cancer and about 19 000 died as a result – if this pattern was to continue, about 85 percent of Canadians diagnosed with lung cancer will die from it. Clearly deaths from lung cancer have *more than doubled* that of both prostate and breast cancers in

Canada. Lung cancer is more preventable than both prostate and breast cancers and the high mortality rate should be a warning for people to stop smoking and to maintain a better quality of life. Some good news was reported in a 2005 by the *Canadian Tobacco Use Monitoring Survey* that in women aged 20 to 24, the percentage of smokers had declined from 30 to 25 percent since 2003 but among teens aged 15 to 19 years, the incidence of smoking still remains unchanged at 18 percent. For men, the incidence of smokers remains unchanged at 31 percent in the Canadian population. There is a need to put more emphasis on educating students in schools about the dangers of cigarette smoke, to promote sensible nutrition and a healthier lifestyle. Teenagers need to know the importance of following a healthier lifestyle and to resist peer pressure. Most smokers start at a younger age and the reported 18 percent of teens as smokers in the Canadian population is exceedingly high and is a health concern. Breaking the smoking habit becomes more difficult later in life and it is important for parents and educators to play a more active role in preventing an addicting habit from starting.

The following comparisons demonstrate the incidence and mortality of prostate in the past ten years and the progress made in detecting, diagnosing and treating cancer. There was an estimated increase of 6 200 new cases of prostate cancer diagnosed from 1994 (14 300) to 2005 (20 500) in Canada. Why was there such a high increase of men being diagnosed with prostate cancer? The reasons include an increasing awareness of men about their health, earlier detection with the DRE and PSA tests and by having a biopsy performed. Why has the mortality rate for prostate cancer been declining and as much as 25 percent over the past ten years? The reasons are *multifold:* more cancers are identified earlier by DRE and PSA tests; doctors monitor their patients and are more aware of the diagnostic tools available; both men and their spouses or partners are becoming more educated about cancer and nutrition; effective curable treatments are available for cancer that is confined to the prostate with earlier detection; and with the information age, prostate support groups and the internet have increased public awareness about prostate cancer. The lifetime probability of dying from prostate cancer is 1 in 26 in Canada. Of all patients diagnosed with prostate cancer after 5 years in Canada, 91 percent of them were still alive.

Between 1991 and 1997, for prostate cancer, "a harvesting effect of the number of incident cases was seen due to unofficial PSA screening…and the age-standardized incidence has recently risen in younger men," as noted by oncologist Pickles and others. Can screening for prostate cancer reduce the mortality rate by identifying cancer earlier? As mentioned earlier, an Ipsos-Reid poll conducted in B.C. found that about 50 percent of men aged 45 to 75 years of age were screened in the past five years with the PSA test for detecting prostate cancer. A study was conducted in the Toronto area and funded by the Canadian Cancer Society (CCS) on PSA screening and the risk of prostate cancer. Dr. Barbara Whylie of the CCS was elated about the results because that study "suggests that early PSA screening may reduce the risk of metastatic prostate cancer." The study was reported in the August 2005 issue of *The Journal of Urology*. A Finnish prostate cancer screening trial of 1 484 men was presented by Dr. Tammela and colleagues in March 2005 at the European Association of Urologists in Istanbul, Turkey. The study suggests that screening increases the possibility for curative treatment of prostate cancer and noted that the proportion of advanced tumours had decreased due to screening. Diagnosing silent cancer by using the serum PSA test increases the stratified incidence of prostate cancer. Perhaps men in British Columbia have the highest incidence of prostate cancer in Canada because of their unofficial screening with the PSA test. Before the PSA era, the annual age-adjusted incidence of prostate cancer rates for Japanese-Americans living in Hawaii and Los Angeles was 48.6 per 100 000 men. From 1988 to 1992, the average incidence rates of prostate cancer for Japanese men in the same regions cited above escalated to 87.6 per 100 000 men. It is interesting to note that in this study by Dr. Shibata and investigators from 1988 to 1992, the average incidence of prostate cancer of native Japanese men was 13.9 per 100 000 men. This data supports a six-fold higher incidence of prostate cancer rates among Japanese-American men as compared with native Japanese men. The age-adjusted mortality rate for prostate cancer for Japanese men in Los Angeles was 9.6 per 100 000 whereas in Japan it was 3.5 per 100 000 men.

Prostate cancer should not be considered as a disease in older men; about 20 percent of this cancer is associated with men who are 65 years of age and younger. The average age when prostate cancer is first diagnosed in men in the U.S. is 69 years. According to Dr. Peter Scardino at Memorial Sloan-Kettering, "Statistically over the lifetime of men over 50

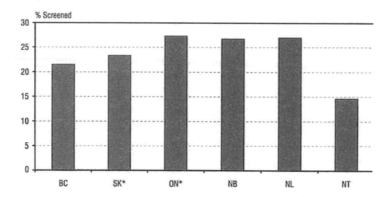

Figure 4.1: Prostate Cancer Screening. Percentage of men aged 40 and over with the PSA test in selected sampling regions in Canada in 2003. From the Canadian Cancer Society and National Cancer Institute of Canada, Canadian Cancer Statistics 2006, Toronto, Canada.

years of age, 42 of every 100 will develop cancer of the prostate, 10 will be diagnosed and 3 will die." Another United States statistic from research conducted by urologist William Catalona a few years ago said that 25 percent of all men *diagnosed* with prostate cancer in the United States would die of the disease. The other 75 percent of men will die *with* their prostate cancer but not from it; the latter statistic has since changed for the better since Dr. Catalona reported it several years ago. In Canada, 20 percent of the men diagnosed with prostate cancer in 2005 will die of the disease and this rate is now comparable to recent U.S. data. *The National Cancer Institute* in the United States and the *Canadian Cancer Society* reported a progressive increase of prostate cancer incidence in all ethnic groups from age 45 to 75 years; men of African descent are at a much greater risk of being diagnosed with prostate cancer while men of Asian descent in North America are at the lowest risk. Recent data on the incidence rate for prostate cancer among white males aged 70 – 74 in North America was 1 041 per 100 000 men, whereas black males for the same age range of 70 – 74 years, the incidence rate was 1 645 per 100 000 men. Clearly, American and Canadian men of African origin are at a much greater risk of being diagnosed with prostate cancer than white males or Asians.

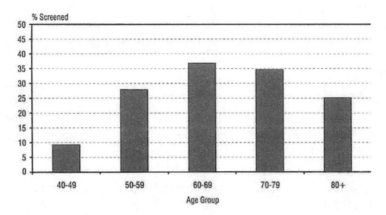

Figure 4.2: Prostate Cancer Screening. Percentage of men aged 40 and over reported screening with the PSA by age group in 2003. From the Canadian Cancer Society and the National Cancer Institute of Canada, *Canadian Cancer Statistics 2006,* Toronto, Canada.

Your Heart or Prostate

You may be asking yourself whether you should see your doctor as soon as possible in view of those seemingly high statistics previously presented about prostate cancer. There is no need to panic but if you are over 40 years of age and have not had a physical examination, book one soon. You may not be too concerned about your prostate condition if less than 40 years of age (unless there is a family history of it) but other areas of concern are your weight or mass, how much and what you eat, your blood pressure, your lipid levels such as cholesterol, low-density lipoproteins (LDL), high-density lipoproteins (HDL), triglycerides and even your glucose level for any suspicious diabetes. Also, monitor your blood chemistry, homocysteine level, as well as thyroid, liver and kidney function. It is important to discuss health concerns, your family history, and possible tests with your family doctor. The International Day for the Evaluation of Abdominal Obesity (IDEA) study of over 170 000 men and women in 63 countries confirms that high waist circumference is associated with cardiovascular disease independent of body mass index (BMI). BMI is an important consideration in cardiovascular disease and diabetes; the website www.bmi-calculator.net can be used to calculate your BMI. The study noted that men with a waist circumference of 94 cm and women who measure 80 cm or more are abdominally obese.

The suggested recommendations for having a PSA test are provided in Chapters 5 and 11. If you smoke, quit because your chances of getting lung cancer and the probability of dying from it will be much higher than from prostate cancer. If you have a family history of prostate cancer or other diseases such as diabetes, then you should have tests done for those concerns. Take the PSA test if a close relative (brother, father, uncle, or grandfather) has been diagnosed with prostate cancer at an early age. As a reminder, if you have not had a physical examination within the last year, book one soon. As mentioned earlier, heart disease and stroke will kill you quicker than prostate cancer. My own prostate cancer was detected as a small tumour during my annual physical examination. My doctor felt a small unusual lump on the right side of the lateral lobe of my prostate after a routine rectal examination about 12 years ago. I did not expect my doctor to discover anything unusual but he discovered that suspicious lump in my prostate gland at an age of 57 years! You should *insist* on having a digital rectal examination or DRE as part of your physical examination especially if you are over the age of 40 years.

Dietary Considerations and Prevention of Prostate Cancer

Nutrition plays an important part in promoting or preventing prostate or breast cancer. Other diseases such as diabetes and cardiovascular problems are also directly related to diet. "For anyone concerned about prostate cancer, a good rule of thumb is to look at what's happening in the world of cardiovascular disease. Ninety-nine times out of 100, what's good for the heart is good for the prostate" as stated by Dr. Peter Grimm of the Seattle Prostate Institute. A diet that features a great deal of red meat, including a high animal fat diet is known to increase the level of cholesterol and also known to promote malignancy of the prostate. Breast cancer incidence also rises with an increase of fat intake. A high fat diet can lead to arteriosclerosis or plaque formation in the arteries that can cause heart attacks that are commonly reported in the North American population. Trans-fatty acids raise LDL cholesterol and lower HDL, the good cholesterol. A 2004 study in the *Journal of Nutrition* stated that heart attack victims had significantly more trans-fats in their fat tissues than did healthy people. Dr. Augustsson and investigators assessed the dietary intake of men and the incidence of prostate cancer using a validated food frequency questionnaire. They found that eating fish more than three times a week was associated with a reduced risk of prostate cancer. It is interesting to note that Japanese men who live in Hawaii are three times as likely to develop prostate cancer than Japanese men living in Nagasaki City, Japan; similarly, Chinese men living in Los Angeles and Vancouver have a five times greater risk of developing prostate cancer than Chinese men living in Singapore or Hong Kong. Dr. Shibata and investigators noted a four-fold to six-fold increase in prostate cancer rates in Japanese-American men in the United States compared with Japanese men in Japan. Prostate cancer is ten times more common in the U.S. and Canada than in Japan. The incidence and mortality rates of prostate cancer are very low among Inuit people living in Greenland. Autopsies conducted between 1990 and 1994 by Canadian and Danish researchers revealed that prostate

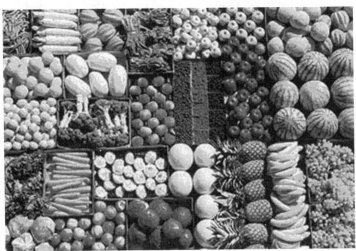

cancer is "rare among the Inuit and that their traditional diet of foods rich in omega-3 polyunsaturated fatty acids" provide that added protection. Diet plays a significant role in promoting or preventing prostate cancer.

The "adult grandchildren of Japanese-Americans develop prostate cancer only slightly less often than the average American man of European descent" concluded Dr. Scardino in his book on *Prostate Cancer.* An *American Cancer Society* survey of 750 000 individuals observed that being obese increased the risk of prostate cancer. Fat consumption correlates significantly with an increased risk of prostate cancer. The survey cited by Dr. Heber was based on per capita of fat consumption among blacks, whites and Asian-Americans and Asian-Canadians living in Los Angeles, San Francisco, Hawaii, Vancouver and Toronto. Dr. Marks and associates at the University of California in Los Angeles investigated the relationship between diet and prostate cancer among native Japanese and second- or third-generation Japanese-American men. The Japanese-American men had more body fat, higher triglyceride and lower estradiol (an estrogen derivative) levels than native Japanese men from Nagoya, Japan. Native Japanese and Japanese-Americans, products of similar genetics but different environments, were shown to have different body compositions that have an influence in advancing the incidence of prostate cancer. A positive statistically significant association of prostate cancer risk and total fat intake was found for all ethnic groups combined. Dr. Heber cited one study conducted by Dr. Giovannucci and investigators and found that more aggressive prostate cancer in patients was significantly correlated with a high fat intake.

Some researchers have found that that the incidence of prostate cancer is increasing in cities like Tokyo, where diets and lifestyles tend to be more westernized. Western fast food is becoming more popular in Asian cities and elsewhere. The size of the prostate gland in men in China is smaller than Chinese men living in Australia after living there for more than 10 years. Genetics did not suddenly increase the size of prostate glands in those Chinese men who migrated and were living in Australia; environment or dietary changes play a significant role by increasing the size of the prostate and changes therein. The lower rate of prostate cancer in Asia is attributed to a lower animal fat consumption and a higher diet of vegetables, soy products, fibre foods containing vitamins A, C, E and beta carotene. Vitamins A, E and beta carotenes are anti-oxidants that *may* provide added protection against epithelial cancers. Drs. Gallagher and Fleshner cautioned that the protective effect of vitamin A and beta-carotene for prostate cancer is lacking at the present time. The county of Qidong in China has the lowest recorded incidence of prostate cancer at 0.5 per 100 000 men in comparison with 121 per 100 000 men in Canada. In a Finnish study of more than 29 000 men noted an incidental and significant finding of linking obesity and prostate cancer. Obese men in that study had a 40 percent risk of developing prostate cancer compared to non-obese men. The same study is discussed in this chapter regarding vitamin E use and the incidence of prostate cancer. Some farmers appear to have an increased risk of developing prostate cancer possibly due to a higher fat intake in their diet and by lengthy exposure to herbicides. In summary, men of Asian origin and living in Asia have a much lower chance of developing prostate cancer than first or second generation Asian-Canadians or Asian-Americans.

Physical activity or exercise is often ignored as a form of therapy and a means of preventing many diseases such as cardiovascular disease, diabetes, stroke, cancers, and respiratory diseases. Dr. D.C. McKenzie, an exercise physiologist at the University of British Columbia, suggests that there is good data to show that regular exercise is associated with prevention of prostate cancer by 10 to 30 percent according to a Stanford study that was reported in a National Cancer Institute article. It should be noted that the biological mechanism to explain the association of exercise and prostate cancer is unknown. Dr. McKenzie explains that being unfit, smoking, having hypertension, a high cholesterol level and being obese will increase the relative risk of mortality. A Dutch study conducted by Dr. Zeegers on the association between physical activity and prostate cancer, found an increased risk of prostate cancer in obese men who were physically active for greater than one hour a day. The latter study of over 58 000 men does not support the hypothesis that physical activity protects men against prostate cancer. Dr. Giovannucci and colleagues, on the other hand, suggest that regular vigorous exercise could slow the progression of prostate cancer especially when there are so many documented benefits of exercise. Dr. Ornish and colleagues in a study reported in *The Journal of Urology* found that intensive lifestyle changes may affect the progression of early prostate cancer. The intensive lifestyle program included a vegan diet supplemented with soy, vitamin E, selenium, vitamin C, moderate exercise, stress management techniques such as yoga and meditation. The mean PSA declined in the experimental group of that study but increased in the control group. A similar study was done by Dr. Ornish and reported in *JAMA* on intensive lifestyle changes on men and women for the reversal of coronary heart disease. Greater regression of coronary atherosclerosis was noted among the experimental group than the control group. The experimental group had a 40 percent reduction in LDL cholesterol level.

The estimated mortality rate in 2005 in the U.S. from prostate cancer per 100 000 men was reported to be 68.1 for African-Americans, 27.7 for white males, and 10.7 for Asian-Americans. In Canada the mortality rate in 2005 for prostate cancer of all ethnic groups was estimated at 26.4 per 100 000 men. The higher prostate cancer death rates among blacks in Africa, the U.S. and Caribbean may be attributed to many factors such as genetic predisposition, diet, lower levels of vitamin D, lack of medical care and the age of men at the time of diagnosis. The importance of vitamin D and ethnic considerations are discussed later in this chapter. Researchers at Children's Hospital in Boston discovered that high blood **cholesterol levels** accelerate the growth of prostate tumours. A high fat diet increases blood cholesterol levels so heed this latest finding on high cholesterol level being linked to the incidence of prostate cancer. Epidemiological studies by Dr. Stamm suggested that people taking cholesterol-lowering drugs like **statins** have a significantly reduced the incidence of prostate and other cancers.

A preliminary Finnish study reported by Dr. Salvatore involving over 29 000 white male smokers aged 50 to 69 years, found that the experimental group of 14 564 men taking 50 milligrams of **vitamin E** (alpha tocopherol) every day for eight years had reduced the incidence of prostate cancer by 32 percent. In addition, there were 41 percent fewer prostate cancer deaths with men taking vitamin E than those not taking it. Be forewarned that the research on taking high amounts of vitamin E supplements is still controversial so get the best advice from your physician before considering this option. Vitamin E acts as a blood thinner as well as an antioxidant. The average intake of vitamin E from the diet of Canadians is about 7 milligrams per day and the recommended daily allowance is 15 milligrams or 22 International Units (IU) – for conversion purposes 100 IU of natural (non-synthetic) vitamin E is equivalent to about 70 milligrams. Almonds, broccoli, spinach, salmon, chickpeas, all-bran cereals contain significant amounts of vitamin E. Most multivitamin supplements contain the amounts of vitamin E that are both effective and safe.

What are the beneficial effects of **selenium**? In a "Johns Hopkins study, men with the lowest level of selenium were those most likely to develop prostate cancer, and men with the highest level of selenium were 50 percent less likely to develop it." Selenium is an essential component of an antioxidant enzyme, glutathione peroxidase and a co-factor in glutathione-S-transferase. Researchers claim that taking selenium with *low* levels of vitamin E is most beneficial in preventing prostate cancer. The recommended daily dose of selenium is 55 micrograms per day. Foods such as meat, tuna, cod, grains, garlic and onions provide the majority of dietary selenium; Brazil nuts are very high in selenium content. Selenium supplements containing more than 200 micrograms may be toxic and are not recommended. Excessive amounts of selenium leads to loss of hair and fingernails, and nausea, fatigue and dizziness. The average intake of selenium for Canadians is about 100 micrograms per day from diet so there is apparently no need to take supplements if you consume the foods mentioned above that contain selenium. Oncologist Strum cited the importance of **boron** in protecting men from prostate cancer. Foods rich in boron include plums, grapes, avocados and nuts such as peanuts and almonds. A study on boron at the Cancer Epidemiology Training Program at UCLA in Los Angeles found that the greater the quantity of boron rich foods consumed, the greater the reduction in risk of being diagnosed with prostate cancer. *Herbicides* are used to kill plant tissues and are known to have an adverse effect on other organisms including humans. U.S. soldiers in Vietnam who had been exposed to Orange Agent, a defoliant also used as a herbicide, suffered from a variety of ailments including cancers. As a precaution, washing of fruits and vegetables are recommended before eating or cooking.

The National Cancer Institute in the U.S. is sponsoring a twelve-year study (a "SELECT" study that translates into "selenium and vitamin E cancer prevention trial") in a population of about 32 400 men in Canada and the U.S. by taking vitamin E alone, selenium alone, vitamin E and selenium and a placebo; the cost this study is 180 million dollars. There are 12 centres in Canada and about 3 000 men are participating in that SELECT study. The scientists will be able to tell which group may develop prostate cancer or which group receives any protective benefits; results will be available in 2012. A large trial of 39 876 healthy women, reported in *Journal of the American Medical Association* (*JAMA*) in July 2005 by Dr. I-Min and colleagues, were randomly assigned to receive 600 IU of Vitamin E on alternate days or to take a placebo and aspirin, or a placebo only. There was no overall benefit for major cardiovascular events or cancer or any decrease in mortality in the health women in the latter study. In a HOPE study that was reported in *JAMA*, "in patients with vascular disease or diabetes mellitus, long-term (6 years) vitamin E supplements of 400 IU per day does not prevent cancer or major cardiovascular events and *may increase the risk for heart failure."* Be cautious when taking high supplements of vitamins and minerals and weigh their benefits and risks. Always check with your physician before taking any supplements, including vitamins.

It may be that dietary fat intake "is promotional rather than causative for development of prostate cancer" as suggested by Dr. Wayne Meikle who has conducted extensive epidemiological studies on prostate cancer in the state of Utah. A diet consisting of broccoli, cauliflower, Brussels sprouts and Swiss chard has anti-cancer properties. Vitamin supplements such as beta carotene or foods high in beta carotene such as the ones mentioned above including yams, beets, lettuce, carrots and tomatoes render some protection against cancer. **Lycopene** is a potent antioxidant and is naturally found in red grapefruits, watermelons, guava, tomato juice, tomato paste and sauce, and berries. A pilot study conducted by Dr. Barber at King's College in London, on 41 men diagnosed with prostate cancer and taking 10 mg of lycopene per day (2 tablets of *Lycoplus)* for 10 months, found that the progression of untreated disease allow extended periods of conservative management of prostate cancer and regression of PSA doubling time. Another study conducted by Dr. Kirsh and investigators, evaluated the association between intake lycopene and tomato products and the risk of prostate cancer. They found that lycopene intake and tomato servings were not associated with prostate cancer risk. One controlled case study carried out by Dr. Qing-Yi Lu and investigators in California noted the relationship between plasma lycopene and other carotenoids and prostate cancer. There was a significant inverse association between plasma lycopene and other carotenoids and prostate cancer. We still do not know for sure of the effectiveness of lycopene in reducing prostate cancer; it is one of the groups of carotenoids and is a potent antioxidant. Further research is needed on lycopene and other antioxidants with the association of prostate cancer risk.

The **soy-based** products such as tofu contain genistein and other isoflavones are antioxidants that clear up free radicals that may reduce the incidence of prostate cancer. Soy also reduces the amount of circulating testosterone and inhibits the enzyme, 5-alpha reductase in the prostate. Soy and isoflavones are phytoestrogens that tend to lower testosterone levels. The latter enzyme helps convert testosterone to dihydrotesterone in the prostate. Dr. Nagata and colleagues in Japan investigated men who consumed 400 millilitres of soymilk daily for eight weeks in a controlled study. They found that serum levels of estrone (one form of estrogen) decreased in the soy supplemented group. There was no difference in free testosterone and estradiol (another form of estrogen) levels between the two groups. Genistein in tofu is known to block the growth of new blood vessels in tumour progression. Tofu, soy protein powder, soy milk, edamame and soy cheese are high in isoflavones. Asian men and women generally include soy products in their diet and probably receive added protection against breast and prostate cancers. There is no proof that soy products prevent prostate cancer. One suggestion is to take vitamin supplements in moderation such as a one-a-day vitamin. Check with your doctor before taking any nutritional and vitamin supplements.

International studies have documented that the average individual consumption of fat for a particular country is related to that country's incidence of prostate cancer. Data strongly suggest that saturated fat consumption in a diet increases the risk of getting prostate cancer. Breast cancer incidence seems to follow the same pattern as prostate cancer with respect to a high fat diet; many trials on diet and incidence of breast cancer are underway in Canada and the United States. One study conducted by Dr. Bairati and colleagues in Quebec and reported in *The Journal of Urology* suggests an association between the consumption of saturated fats and prostate cancer progression. Patients in the study were treated with surgery or radiotherapy and included 142 patients with advanced prostate cancer and 242 with local stages of cancer. A positive trend on prostate cancer progression was observed in patients for total animal fat intake while a negative trend was noted in patients for vegetable fat intake. Dr. Peter Carroll reported that obese men are more likely to have positive surgical margins; he also stated that although diet and supplements may reduce the risk of prostate cancer, it is unknown whether they have any effect in men already diagnosed. In an animal study, a high fat diet fed to genetically engineered mice resulted in enlarged prostate glands, obesity and prostate cancer. The control group of mice had pea size prostate glands, showed no obesity, and no prostate cancer. The research was conducted by Dr. Neil Fleshner and colleagues at Princess Margaret Hospital in Toronto. A large study of more than 900 000 U.S. adults was conducted by Dr. Calle and other investigators to examine body weight or mass and the risk of death from cancers. Body mass index (BMI) is the weight in kilograms divided by the square of the height in metres. In both sexes, higher BMI was significantly associated with higher death rates due to cancer of the esophagus, colon, rectum, liver, gall bladder, pancreas, kidney and stomach. In women, increased death rates with higher BMI were noted for cancers of the breast, uterus, cervix and ovaries. In men with higher BMI, there was an increase rate in prostate cancer. Type II diabetes is associated with obesity so it is wise to check your BMI level and keep within the acceptable range. You may check your BMI at the website: www.bmi-calculator.net. As mentioned earlier, increasing waist circumference is a factor for promoting cardiovascular disease. What is good for the heart is also good for the prostate.

It is well known that antioxidants suppress mutations on DNA thereby reducing the incidence of many cancers. Antioxidants are substances that protect the DNA and cells from damage caused by free radicals or unstable molecules. Polyphenols in green tea may hold some promise acting as antioxidants and cancer-inhibiting agents; more research is needed to prove that green tea reduces the incidence of prostate cancer. Green tea is a good source of vitamin K needed in blood clotting mechanisms. In a study in China and carried out by the U.S. *National Cancer Institute,* researchers found that "900 patients with esophageal cancer when compared with 1 500 healthy people, and looking at the patients who did not smoke or drink alcohol, the tea drinkers were about 60 percent less likely to develop cancer than others." A Cornell University study suggest that eating an apple a day gives your body more antioxidants and cancer fighting properties than taking vitamin supplements – eating a fresh apple and its skin is equivalent to the antioxidants in 1500 milligrams of vitamin C. Eating a variety of fruits and vegetables may provide the necessary vitamins and antioxidants that would reduce the need to take vitamin supplements. Plant products contain very many protective phytochemicals that scientists have not yet isolated or analyzed for anti-carcinogenic properties so eating more vegetables and fruits would do more good than harm. As an additional protection, a one-a-day vitamin/mineral supplement may be taken with a balanced dietary intake and with the advice of your physician. The Canadian Cancer Society (CCS) has published a booklet entitled "Eat Well, Be Alive" and provides food tips and recipes. "Eating well, being active and staying at a healthy weight are among the best ways to reduce your risk of cancer" is one of its conclusions. So as to guide you in making any decision about dietary supplements, you may access the Quackwatch website at www.quackwatch.org for another opinion. The mission of that website is to inform the public of health-related frauds, myth, fad and fallacies.

Family History

Family history and genetics play significant roles in understanding how a disease or disorder progresses from one generation to the next. Refer to the information presented in Chapters 1 and 2 with regard to specific genes for prostate cancer susceptibility on chromosomes 1, 4, 5, 7, 8, 16, 19, 20, and the X and Y chromosomes, as well as the p53 gene that, when mutated, would trigger changes in the DNA and promote abnormal cell growth. Scientists are interested in studying close relatives such as brothers and sisters, mothers and fathers, uncles and aunts and the incidence of cancers using an entire family tree. "A three-fold increase in risk has been observed in men whose brothers and father have prostate cancer" concluded Dr. Meikle in a Utah data base study of 2 824 prostate cancer cases. "The relative risk for all sites (prostate and other cancers) for brothers of the cases (of prostate cancer) was 1.6, whereas it was 2.2 for a brother whose sister had breast cancer." If the two first-degree relatives have prostate cancer, then the risk of another family member, such as a father, brother or son getting cancer, will be greater. Dr. Verhage and colleagues in the Netherlands found that prostate cancer has a 2.9-fold increased risk for first-degree relatives. The familial risk for prostate cancer was surprisingly higher among brothers as compared with fathers. The National Cancer Institute (NCI) in the U.S reported that approximately 9.6 percent of an Iowa cohort had a family history of breast and/or ovarian cancer sister at baseline, and this was positively associated with prostate cancer risk. Dr. Hemminki, using a Swedish Family-Cancer Database, found that the standardized incidence ratios for prostate cancer were increased in sons when mothers were diagnosed with breast and ovarian cancers. A report by Dr. Kirchhoff and colleagues analyzed the blood from 251 Ashkenazi men with prostate cancer together with 1472 Ashkenazi male volunteers without prostate cancer. They found that the mutation of the breast cancer gene BRCA2 had an increased risk of prostate cancer developing in the cancer subjects studied. Since a man carries half of his mother's genes that can also mutate, you could therefore hypothesize that a mutation on the breast cancer gene (BRCA2) is associated with an increased risk of prostate cancer.

One should also note that the younger the family member is when he is diagnosed, the greater are the chances of his brother or his son getting prostate cancer. Brothers and sons of women who have had breast cancer or carry a mutant form of genes linked to breast and prostate cancer have a somewhat elevated risk of developing prostate cancer according to Drs. Granick and Fair. It does not follow that if one brother gets prostate cancer that the other one will have an equal risk of getting the disease. Urologist Scardino reported that one of his patients diagnosed with prostate cancer at an age of 62 years he had three sons in their thirties and who were all diagnosed with prostate cancer. The National Cancer Institute reported that 5 to 10 percent of prostate cancer cases are believed to be due primarily to high-risk inherited factors of prostate cancer susceptibility genes. The Urological Research Foundation in the U.S. headed by Dr. Catalona is investigating family links and studied more than 500 brothers from over 200 families to determine if brothers with prostate cancer share markers more often than expected, that is, more than 50 percent of the time. If sharing of markers is found then gene identification for prostate cancer susceptibility could possibly be investigated further. Oncologist Strum reported that "approximately one in four men diagnosed with prostate cancer will demonstrate evidence of genetic clustering of prostate cancer...and 19 % are considered to be cases of hereditary prostate cancer whereas 81 % are designated as having familial prostate cancer." *Familial prostate cancer* refers to clustering of cancers in families while *hereditary prostate cancer* is characterized by transmission of a single gene from father to son, or from father to daughter and then to a grandson.

The genetic markers on chromosomes 1, 4, 5, 8, 7, 16, 19, 20 and the X and Y chromosome are implicated in triggering prostate cancer when the gene expression is lost or becomes mutated. Chromosome 16 carries a tumour suppressor gene and when mutated or through loss of expression has shown to be a strong linkage with prostate cancer. A tumour suppressor gene is a gene whose loss of function contributes to the development of cancer. Mutations in the p53 tumour suppressor gene are "generally believed to be a late event in the progression of prostate cancer..." according to Dr. Downing. At the Marshfield Medical Research Foundation in

Wisconsin, researchers are mapping chromosomes 1, 4, 5, 7, 8, 11, 16 and 19 that might harbour genes that predispose men to prostate cancer and tumour growth. Researchers noted that regions of chromosomes 7 and 19 are linked with "aggressive forms of prostate cancer." A report from Sweden in the journal *Urology* concluded that "hereditary susceptibility is now considered the strongest risk for prostate cancer and has profound clinical importance." One large cohort study by Dr. Lichtenstein and colleagues reported in the *New England Journal of Medicine* that "statistically significant effects of heritable factors were observed for prostate cancer." The investigators also noted that "the relatively large effect of heritability in cancer at a few sites (such as prostate and colorectal cancer) suggests major gaps in our knowledge of the genetics of cancer." Dr. Strum listed three criteria to designate a patient as having hereditary prostate cancer: "a family with three generations affected by prostate cancer; three first-degree relatives affected (brothers/father); and two relatives affected before the age of 55 years." Drs. Walsh and Partin noted that prostate carcinoma may be inherited as an automosal dominant trait; it is estimated to be associated with 43 percent of men when diagnosis was made at an age of less than 55 years. Epidemiological studies conducted by Dr. Bratt and investigators indicate that dominantly inherited susceptibility genes cause 5 to 10 percent of all prostate cancer cases and as much as 30 to 40 percent of early onset disease.

In the future, identifying prostate cancer genes and knowing their specific gene loci will become potential clinical markers for prostate cancer. More research is needed to determine specific genetic links with prostate cancer which may lead to better treatments involving genetics. As mentioned in Chapter 2, the gene identified as PCA3 is expressed in prostate cancer provides evidence of the new urine-based genetic test known as uPM3 for detecting prostate cancer with high accuracy. Gene technology in the future will unravel some of the mysteries scientists struggle with today. Gene chips or DNA chips carry thousands of genetic information. The hope is that it will be possible for these devices to diagnose diseases with a genetic base or to discover a treatment for a particular genetic disease. **Gene chips** will identify who is at risk of a disease. But the big question still remains, would the individual want to know his genetic expressions, those hidden genes that normally pose no real or immediate health problems?

Ethnic Considerations

Earlier the link of the high incidence of prostate cancer was discussed among the men of African or Afro-Caribbean origin in the Canadian and American population. Ethnic differences play an important role in the incidence of prostate cancer in addition to dietary factors. The black population including African-Americans and African-Canadians, Caribbean blacks and especially Jamaicans, demonstrate an increased risk of developing prostate cancer. The highest incidence of prostate cancer was reportedly found to be in Kingston, Jamaica – an average of 304 per 100 000 men in Kingston. The age-adjusted prostate cancer cases diagnosed among men of African origin are significantly higher than white Canadian or American males; the age-standardized incidence rate among Canadian men in 2006 is estimated to be 121 per 100 000 men. One screening study was conducted in the island of Tobago in the Caribbean on an Afro-Caribbean population of 2 484 males aged 40 to 79 years. PSA and DRE were determined in the sample population. Men with a PSA of 4 ng/ml or greater and/or with an abnormal DRE had biopsies performed. The screening results indicated a very high prevalence of prostate cancer in Afro-Caribbean males. The data from the study supports the hypothesis that genetics and/or environmental factors contribute to the high incidence of prostate cancer in Tobago among men of African descent. The mortality rate among African-Americans is more than twice as high as in Caucasians in the United States. Why do men of darker skin have a higher risk of developing prostate cancer? One explanation might be that in the United States, and elsewhere, black men do not have the same access to medical care as white males and it is often too late when a diagnosis is made. We do not have all the answers for ethnic differences but genetics play a role or genetic susceptibility of a set of factors play some part. Another reason for differences in prostate cancer susceptibility for black men versus white men points to insufficient intake of vitamin D among people of black skin. The role of **Vitamin D** as an antioxidant and protection against prostate cancer is discussed later in this chapter.

Serum testosterone concentration appears to be higher in black men than in white men, particularly at a younger age according to Dr. Gapstur and investigators in an article in the journal *Cancer Epidemiology Biomarkers & Prevention*. The investigators also noted that increasing obesity in the abdominal area is associated with decreasing total testosterone and sex hormone-binding globulin levels in white and black men. Dr. Scardino notes that young African-American men tend to have higher levels of prostate cancer-promoting testosterone than whites or Asians – that small amount of testosterone that targets the prostate gland. New light has been shed on the receptors of testosterone in prostate cells among ethnic groups – the genetic carriers of testosterone into cells. Protein receptors tag onto hormones and exert their effect on cells including prostate and muscle cells. In Asians, the length of the receptor for testosterone is large; it is intermediate in size in white men while short receptors are present in black men. The shorter the receptor, the more efficient it is for testosterone to pass into prostate cells – a greater amount of testosterone therefore passes into the prostate gland in a given time in black men than for white or Asian men. A greater supply of testosterone in the prostate increases the activity of cellular function. This may be another reason why men of African origin are more susceptible to getting prostate cancer by having a more efficient way for testosterone to pass into the prostate gland. One should note that the testosterone receptor is a protein which has a genetic origin like all proteins. Asians are at the lowest risk of having the hormone testosterone passing into the prostate gland. But this genetic susceptibility is only part of the equation why African-Canadian and American men are at a greater risk of getting prostate cancer. A recent study conducted by Dr. Severi and investigators on circulating steroid hormones and the risk of prostate cancer failed to support the hypothesis that circulating androgens are positively associated with prostate cancer risk. Dr. Severi said that "high testosterone and adrenal androgens are associated with reduced risk of aggressive prostate cancer but not with aggressive disease."

Vitamin D is known to protect against prostate cancer by keeping cells well differentiated by maintaining their shape and keeping cells intact. The research by Dr. Oakley-Girvan and collaborators linked an early onset of prostate cancer and vitamin D receptor. There is some correlation between the lack of vitamin D and the incidence of prostate cancer. Vitamin D inhibits prostate cancer cell growth, angiogenesis and metastases. The action of vitamin D is mediated by a receptor. The hormonally active form of vitamin D known as 1,2,5-dihydroxyvitamin D, is responsible for inhibiting cancer cell growth and prevents new growth of blood vessels (angiogenesis) that cancer cells need for their growth. Vitamin D levels in humans increase in the presence of sunlight. Because black skin is more efficient at blocking out sunlight, black men are known to have lower levels of vitamin D, making them more susceptible to prostate cancer. One study compared the composition of blood vitamin D levels of black men living in Zaire, Africa, with their counterparts in Belgium. The study found a lower level of vitamin D in those former Zairian men living in Belgium, a northern region that receives less sunlight than Zaire. Men of African ancestry in regions with less sunlight are at a greater risk of developing prostate cancer. Men who are at risk should take a multivitamin supplement containing 400 IU of vitamin D and more during the winter months in North America or in Europe. The average vitamin D intake among North Americans aged 50 or older is only 5 micrograms per day, half of what is considered adequate intake.

You often hear the expression, "You are what you eat." Many North Americans and Europeans of all ethnic groups collectively consume too much meat and animal fat in their diet compared with Asians. Are North Americans eating too many hamburgers, fried foods including chicken (with its skin included for taste), French fries, and not enough fruit and vegetables? Dr. Rodriguez and associates at the Epidemiology and Surveillance Research in Atlanta, U.S.A., examined the association of red meat intake and the risk of prostate cancer among black and white males. They excluded men with a history of cancer and incomplete dietary information. The researchers discovered that among black men the total red meat intake (processed and unprocessed) was associated with a higher risk of prostate cancer than in white men. The processed meats included sausages, bacon and hot dogs. A prolonged diet low in fat and high in fibre would eventually result in lowering the level of blood cholesterol. As mentioned earlier, a diet high in animal fats or saturated fats will elevate blood cholesterol levels. High cholesterol levels are known to accelerate the growth of prostate tumours as reported in a *Journal of Clinical Investigation* article from the research at Children's Hospital in Boston. Lowering cholesterol levels from diet and by men using cholesterol-lowering drugs such as statins have significantly reduced the risk of prostate cancer. "There is increasing evidence that statins are synergistic with other chemopreventive agents" concluded Dr. Stamm in one study. Dr. Platz at Johns Hopkins and investigators at the NIH followed over 34 000 men who reported on their use of cholesterol-lowering drugs. They found that men taking statins had a 54 percent lower risk of advanced prostate cancers than those not taking those drugs. As urologist Scardino stated "the best way we know is to live a heart-healthy lifestyle" for reducing the incidence of prostate cancer.

A study conducted by Dr. Iona Cheng and investigators compared the PSA and hormone levels among men in Singapore and the United States. None of the men had a history of prostate cancer when blood samples were taken and analyzed in the same laboratory. PSA and testosterone levels in Chinese men in Singapore, African-Americans, U.S. whites, Japanese Americans and U.S. Latinos were recorded. One significant finding was that the PSA levels in Singapore Chinese men *were higher* than in U.S. white, U.S. Latino and Japanese-Americans. In fact, Singapore Chinese men at ages 45 to 64 had *higher* PSA levels than men at the ages of 65 to 74 years. In that study, researchers found that testosterone levels did not reflect ethnic patterns of disease. Since the incidence rate of prostate cancer is higher in the United States than in Singapore, the PSA test may be a poor marker of prostate cancer in the low risk group of men from Singapore. *PSA levels therefore failed to correlate with the low prostate cancer incidence and mortality rates in Singapore.* The authors of the study also indicated that the incidence and mortality rates of prostate cancer in Singapore seem to be on the increase.

Other Risk Factors

Dr. Wen-Hsiang and other researchers at the Johns Hopkins Oncology Centre isolated an enzyme known as glutathione S-transferase that was missing in 88 of the 91 human prostate cancers, after examining tissues of patients and autopsies. Genes control the synthesis of enzymes and proteins and more information about prostatic proteins and enzymes as genetic markers of the prostate cancer will emerge. Several genes are responsible for promoting prostate cancer; the Genome Project, Celera Genomics and other research centres that are continuing their work will discover many more genetic markers for prostate cancer and other cancers. Is there a built-in switch to turn on the prostate specific antigen enzyme which is a marker for prostate problems, including cancer? Would the specific prostate cancer genes identified on chromosomes be helpful in the early diagnosis of prostate cancer, and if so, will men opt for earlier treatment even when no cancer is detected? Ethical issues may become a challenge for women who may learn that they carry the breast cancer genes and are forced to decide to seek treatment in order to avoid getting cancer later in life.

Researchers at the University of North Carolina investigated the influence of **ultraviolet radiation** (UV) as a factor in promoting prostate cancer. Drs. Bodiwala and Strange at Staffordshire, England, described a study with 212 prostate cancer men and 135 men with BPH. The investigators used a validated questionnaire to obtain data in their study. They found that higher levels of exposure to UV radiation were significantly associated with a reduced risk of prostate cancer. There may be some evidence to demonstrate that an increasing amount of ultraviolet radiation may *protect* a person from getting prostate cancer. In countries like Sweden, Denmark, Canada and Iceland where the incidence of prostate cancer appears to be the highest among the global white population, the exposure rate to ultraviolet light is the lowest. The researchers also indicated that African-American men absorb less ultraviolet light and together with lower levels of vitamin D, contribute to an increased risk of prostate cancer. Can ultraviolet light also be an additional factor which promotes prostate cancer among men of dark skin and white males living in northern regions? More research is definitely required to understand the role played by ultraviolet light. I question how valid an association with ultraviolet light and prostate cancer could be considered when other factors including vitamin D and sunlight come into the equation and are inseparable!

Another concern that has been under investigation is whether having a vasectomy can promote the incidence of prostate cancer. Studies show that men who had **vasectomy** procedures have *no definite link* with an increase in the rate of prostatic cancer compared with non-vasectomy individuals, despite a study reported by Dr. Edward Giovannucci in 1993 that apparently shows a link. Conclusions regarding causality between vasectomy and prostate cancer are *not* valid as reported in *Journal of the American Medical Association* as well as from other sources; the latter article in *JAMA* questioned some of the procedures and findings of Giovannucci. "There are two other published cohort studies which show no statistically significantly increased risk of prostate cancer following vasectomy" according to the UBC Prostate Clinic Fax Line. What about smoking and the incidence of prostate cancer? Dr. Janet Stanford at the Seattle *Hutchison Cancer Research Center* in a study found that men under the age of 65 years and who had a history of **smoking** a pack of cigarettes a day for 40 years or two packs for 20 years "face twice the risk of developing more aggressive forms of prostate cancer than men who have not smoked." The study involved more than 1 450 Seattle-area men 40 to 66 years of age. Dr. Stanford speculated that smoking can increase the circulating androgens as well as the presence of cadmium in cigarettes that is weakly linked to prostate cancer. Cancers associated with heavy smokers include lung, bladder, cervix, esophagus and kidney.

Dr. Stanford and colleagues also found that "men who consume four or more glasses of **red wine** per week reduced their risk of prostate cancer by 50 percent." Red wine, but not white wine, beer or hard spirits contains a substance known as resveratrol which is an antioxidant that enhances apoptosis (suicide of cells), and may also act as a mild estrogen. A study in Italy by Dr. Sgambato and colleagues noted that resveratrol is a naturally occurring phenolic compound and acts as an antimutagenic/anticarcinogenic agent by preventing oxidative DNA damage. Dr. Stanford suggests consuming "four to eight 4-ounce drinks of red wine per week" is adequate. Some people believe that zinc is good for the prostate. The prostate accumulates more zinc than any other part of the body but using zinc as a supplement for prostate health and prevention of cancer or BPH is not recommended. An article in the *Journal of the National Cancer Institute* noted that men who take more than 100 mg of zinc a day may actually double their risk of advanced prostate cancer. Men who took zinc supplements for 10 years or more also doubled their risk of having prostate cancer. Although zinc is found in the prostate, it does not follow that high zinc supplements for prostate health is recommended. **Serum insulin growth factor-1** (IGF-1) at higher levels has been associated with an increased risk for later development of prostate cancer. The research conducted by Dr. Nam and investigators in Canada measured IGF-1 levels in men with high–grade prostatic intraepithelial neoplasia (HGPIN) together with controls. The levels of blood IGF-1 were significantly higher in men with HGPIN as compared with the controls. High serum IGF-1 levels appear to demonstrate a risk factor but it is not a tumour marker for prostate cancer. The researchers also noted that patients with HGPIN are 30 to 50 percent more likely to develop prostate cancer.

The Canadian Cancer Society (CCS) has issued a prevention strategy and statement to all Canadians with suggestions on ways to control the risks of developing cancer. Cancer is the leading cause of premature death in Canada and seems to be the most feared disease. One in three Canadians develops cancer; the good news is that one half of those cancer cases diagnosed will become long-term survivors. Due to an aging population and population growth, "the incidence of cancer in Canada will likely increase by as much as 70% over the next 15 years," claims the CCS report. The CCS acknowledges that at least 50 percent of cancer cases can be prevented through "healthy living, public policies and systemic changes that protect the health of Canadians." Not smoking, avoiding second-hand smoke, eating well, exercising regularly, and practicing sun protection are some key steps in reducing your cancer risk. *Statistics Canada* reported that 25 percent of Canadian adults are at a weight that negatively affects their health.

This information on detection, diagnosis and treatment options for prostate cancer, or any suggestions relating to diet, vitamins or dietary supplements are not intended to replace the advice of doctors and other health-care professionals. Each individual case is unique and this book offers no medical advice on any individual situation. The opinions expressed throughout this book represent my personal views and from the research cited in the literature. With new research on prostate cancer emerging weekly in the literature, some of the new information presented today will likely change the way cancer is treated or detected.

Chapter 5
Detecting and Diagnosing Prostate Cancer

By reading this chapter you will learn:

- The importance and limitations of the digital rectal examination.

- How is the DRE done?

- What is the PSA, its role in screening and importance in diagnosis?

- Limitations and confusion about the total PSA test.

- False negative and false positive PSA.

- Your age, PSA level and risk of being diagnosed with prostate cancer.

- When to test or retest with the PSA?

- The PSA velocity and doubling time in detecting disease.

- The free serum PSA, pro-PSA, and the uPM3 urine test or prostate cancer detection.

- How is a biopsy done?

- When is a biopsy recommended for specific PSA values?

- What does the research say about PSA cutoff values for a biopsy?

The Digital Rectal Exam

The most appropriate initial tests available for prostate cancer detection or benign prostate hypertrophy (BPH) is the **digital rectal examination** (DRE) performed by your general practitioner or urologist, followed by a **prostate specific antigen** (PSA) test. To conduct a DRE the physician inserts a lubricated gloved finger into the rectum and feels the wall of the prostate gland. The entire prostate gland cannot be felt by this means; none of the transition zone and regions at the front or anterior of the gland is palpable. The part that is readily felt by DRE is closest to the rectal wall and the lateral regions of the peripheral zone. Fortunately, the peripheral zone is the site of most prostate cancer tumours. Any abnormal firmness or hard nodule is a possible indication of cancer and further evaluation will be necessary. A nodule in the prostate does not necessarily confirm the presence of cancer although the normal prostate is relatively soft or spongy. Your primary care physician will refer you to an urologist if something is abnormal in the DRE test. Before going to see an urologist or oncologist your physician should order a PSA test. Cancer may be present at an early stage since tumours are much too small to be felt by DRE and are only visible by microscopic examination. Many cancers are multifocal and present as tiny tumours throughout the gland that may pose no immediate risk. Cancer in the transition zone is almost never felt by DRE although about 20 percent of prostate cancer occurs in this area. The DRE is an initial test for detecting prostate cancer but it is not meant to confirm or negate malignancy.

The DRE is performed in a variety of ways by the patient assuming different body positions so as to enable the physician to examine as much of the prostate gland as possible. I am more comfortable when my general practitioner has me to lie on my side on the examination table. My urologist had me lie on my back with my legs raised but with my feet kept flat on the examining table. Another position that some physicians use for DRE is for the patient to bend over the edge of the examining table while standing. Good doctors know how to put the patient at ease so he does not have to feel that the procedure is dehumanizing and it should not be done in a rough manner. A soft touch is required to detect suspicious lumps.

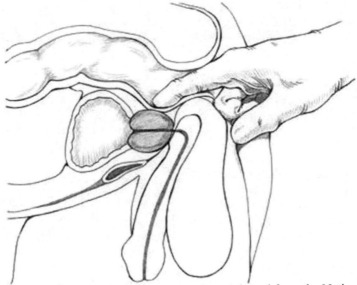

Figure 5.1: Digital rectal examination procedure. Adapted from the National Kidney and Urologic Diseases Information Clearinghouse, National Institute of Health.

Ask your doctor in advance how the digital exam is done if she/he has not already informed you. Your buttocks muscles should be completely relaxed. Be forewarned that the DRE is a subjective test and some physicians could make a decision that is not correct. Urologists are better trained than general practitioners in performing the DRE and in making an appropriate decision. In combination with the results from the PSA test, sound decisions can be made on a man's prostate condition before any biopsy is done. A DRE should be part of your annual physical examination.

One study conducted by Dr. Philip and colleagues in England when the DRE was performed in the diagnosis and clinical staging of early prostate cancer concluded that "of the 196 patients with abnormal DRE, 47 percent had cancer on biopsy; in patients with normal DRE, 59 cancers were detected." There was no correlation between the DRE, biopsy findings as well as pathological staging of prostate cancer from the latter study in the *British Journal of Urology International.* The DRE in that study did not identify patients who had prostate cancer but DRE still has an important place in assessing patients with prostate conditions. Prostate cancer is not confined to one section of glandular tissue as several sites of early malignancy are commonly found – many cancers are multifocal. Generally, the DRE should be followed up by a PSA test in men over 45 years of age if there is a family history of prostate cancer and for all men over 50 years of age. You may refer to the suggested recommendations for having a PSA test in the population as discussed by various organizations and associations in the U.S. and Canada in this chapter and in Chapter 11.

Prostate Specific Antigen Test

Prostate specific antigen (PSA) is synthesized in the prostate gland and consists of a glycoprotein comprising of 237 amino acid residues and 8 percent carbohydrate. PSA levels are high in seminal fluid that makes up the semen in ejaculate. PSA molecule synthesized in the prostate diffuses into the blood and is present in the serum component; you may hear the term *serum PSA* when the doctor orders a test for you. The PSA test was first discovered in 1979 and the U.S. Food and Drug Administration (FDA) approved a Hybritech PSA test in 1985 to track recurrent prostate cancer but it was not initially meant as a test for detecting prostate cancer. Because PSA is a protein substance, the gene that encodes it was found to be on chromosome number 19 – genes are responsible for the synthesis of proteins. PSA as a screening test for prostate cancer began in 1986 in the U.S. after receiving approval by the U.S. Food and Drug Administration. Dr. Ming Chu is one of the pioneering researchers of the PSA test. Some researchers were critical of the way clinicians used the PSA test; one earlier comment suggested it was a disaster for the health-care system, referring to the way the test was being used or even abused. In 1983, Dr. Ming Wang and colleagues undertook the purification of the PSA test. Today the controversy still persists as to whether PSA screening should be open to men in their forties or for men with no prostate symptoms. By definition, *screening* refers to the use of a test with a person who appears well in order to detect a disease at an early stage. Undiagnosed and fit men or those with no suspicion of prostate problems should understand the implications of the PSA test. A survey conducted by an Ipsos-Reid poll in British Columbia found that 50 percent of men aged 45-75 had been screened in the past five years with the PSA test. Dr. Hugosson and colleagues in a Swedish study of 9 972 men from 50 to 65 years of age who were randomized to PSA screening concluded that in men with a PSA of less than 2 ng/ml, it seems safe to offer repeat screening after two years with PSA only. Men with a PSA of 2 to 3 ng/ml or greater than 3 ng/ml with a negative biopsy should be screened earlier or more often than every two years according to that study.

In Canada, early detection of prostate cancer has been increasing within the past ten years and the mortality rate has fortunately been declining. In my opinion, earlier detection of prostate cancer with PSA testing, diagnosis and appropriate treatment has saved lives. Even though PSA screening by itself has not been conclusively demonstrated to reduce the mortality rate of prostate cancer, it appears that PSA testing leads to earlier treatment, especially in younger men. A preliminary Finnish study of 32 000 men investigated by Dr. Tammela and colleagues suggested that screening increases the possibility for curative treatment of prostate cancer and noted that the proportion of advanced tumours have declined. Doctors and patients accept the fact that PSA testing results in early detection of prostate cancer before it becomes a disease that is untreatable. Incidentally, nine out of ten urologists in Ontario always or often screen men using the PSA test, according to an Ipsos-Reid survey. "In 2001 approximately 75 % of men in the U.S. of 50 years and older have reported PSA screening and 54 % have reported regular PSA screening" according to the research conducted by Dr. Ian Thompson.

The physiology of the PSA is not well known but it is believed to have a protease or enzyme activity and plays an important role in the liquefaction of the seminal fluid – the fluid that is part of semen synthesized and secreted from the prostate gland and seminal vesicles. The DRE by itself is not sensitive enough to detect small tumours especially in stage A cancer or at any early stage. If early cancer is present it will be at the microscopic level and discovered through a biopsy in stage A or T1a to T1c (the TNM system); staging systems are explained in Chapter 6. Most cancers are found at an early stage even when the DRE is negative and when men experience BPH symptoms. The PSA test is the best test available to assess the activity of the prostate and for detecting prostate cancer but the value or level established has its limitations; there is still some uncertainty as to how the test is being interpreted. The PSA reading is not always 100 percent reliable in detecting the presence of prostate cancer, especially when the cancer is well differentiated, microscopic or even with small palpable tumours. More than 50 percent of men with elevated PSA levels are known to be cancer-free. In recent years more doctors are recommending that their patients take the PSA test and more patients are also asking for it. Urologist Goldenberg and his team of researchers at the Vancouver Prostate Clinic stated: "There is accumulating evidence to suggest that when used as a screening tool in the appropriate population, serum PSA is the single best test for early detection of prostate cancer and compares favorably with screening tests for breast and cervical cancers." There should be unanimous agreement with the latter statement. In addition to the total serum PSA test, some newer tests have been developed; these are the free PSA, pro-PSA and the recent urine-based uPM3 test that seem to be meaningful diagnostic tools used in conjunction with the total PSA test. Assays are now available that specifically measure the free and complexed PSA isoforms. The FDA has approved both the free and complex PSA tests. The free PSA test is also approved in Canada. When the total PSA is taken it includes both the free and bound isoforms.

Of course, a man over the age of 40 years without any prostate problems and with no family history of prostate diseases could request a PSA test but he may still have to pay for it in some provinces in Canada. However, if the physician has reason to believe that a PSA is warranted, the patient is not required to pay for the test. Men whose PSA values are suspiciously high for their age should be re-evaluated months later; in fact about six months to ten months later, another PSA test is recommended to determine the velocity of the PSA, how much it has risen if at all. The combination of the PSA velocity and doubling time, a man's PSA value, DRE, and Gleason grade after a biopsy are generally used to determine if cancer is present and how aggressive the tumour(s) may be. Your physician will recommend biopsy if the PSA doubling time, velocity or PSA level are a concern. An editorial in *The Journal of Urology* in 2005 and the Canadian Cancer Society noted that the mortality rate for prostate cancer has been decreasing in the U.S. and Canada and that it is probably due to due early detection of cancer and curative treatment with modern therapies. More men in Canada and the U.S. are being diagnosed at an earlier age for prostate cancer. In most of those cases diagnosed, prostate cancer tumours are smaller, multifocal, of lower stage and grade, and amenable to curative treatment. The editorial noted that "approximately 90% of prostate cancers detected today are clinically localized...and we should begin by unlinking detection and treatment, as they are separate processes." Once prostate cancer is detected and localized, the level of treatment, aggressive or conservative, is decided after a consultation between the patient and his physician. A man's age and health at the time of diagnosis are important factors in deciding on the kind of treatment options.

PSA Values, Cutoffs and Persistent Uncertainty

A PSA level above 4 microgram per litre (ug/l) is suspicious of malignancy of the prostate and can be confirmed by a needle biopsy sample. There are known cases of *false negatives* with the total PSA test in any given population at a level where cancer should not be normally present. The level of the PSA value may be as low as 0.2 ug/l, as it was in my situation, and the individual could still test positive for cancer by microscopic investigation with biopsy samples; my DRE presented a small, palpable tumour. Dr. Thompson and other investigators in a study with 2 950 men from 62 to 91 years of age discovered that the "prevalence of prostate cancer was 6.6% among men with a PSA level of 0.5 ng/ml and lower, and 10.1% among those with PSA values of 0.6 to 1.0 ng/ml...and biopsy detected prostate cancer including high-grade cancers, is not rare among men with PSA levels of 4.0 ng/ml or less." Urologist Thompson summarized that an unusually high percent of men in the population with a PSA less than 4.0 ng/ml are known to have prostate cancer. Small tumours, palpable or not, may not elevate PSA values. Indeed many cancers are multifocal or present in several sites within the prostate gland, are small and may be missed by ultrasound on biopsy. Dr. Patrick Walsh and others noted that about 25 percent of men with prostate cancer have low PSA values, that is, nothing looks suspicious about the PSA values. Dr. Scardino cautioned that "in rare cases high grade cancer functions so abnormally that cells ironically make very little PSA." On the other hand, an individual may *not* have a cancerous tumour but gets a high PSA reading (between 4 ug/l and 10 ug/l), or a *false positive* for prostate cancer; the latter is especially common in men with BPH, prostatitis or in some men over the age of 70 years when no cancer is present. You should be also aware of the latter conditions including inflammation in the prostate gland, the presence of larger cancerous tumours, and a higher grade of tumour could result in an elevated PSA value. The National Institute of Health reported that 25 to 30 percent of men who have a biopsy due to elevated PSA levels actually have prostate cancer. Urologists and oncologists understand that the PSA can also fluctuate from day to day but a continuous rise over a few months needs attention. As a reminder, the PSA test by itself cannot confirm the presence of cancer; cancer may be highly suspicious if the PSA level is elevated or the PSA doubling time occurs in less than one year. Later in this chapter the PSA velocity and doubling time will be discussed.

An individual may be alarmed by having high a PSA reading and could agonize that he may perhaps have prostate cancer, causing him to needlessly worry until a biopsy is performed. Patients and physicians should be aware of false readings (positive or negative) in a significant number of cases. "Rates of false-positive PSA screening test results increase with advancing of age.... It should be remembered that PSA testing is meant to assess risk and not to diagnose cancer. An elevated PSA reading does not mean the presence of cancer but rather indicates the presence of prostatic disease and the need for further evaluation," according to noted urologist William Catalona in an article in the *Journal of the American Medical Association* (*JAMA*). Dr. Catalona also cautions that "cancers smaller than 1 cubic centimetre usually do not elevate PSA levels, whereas those larger than this usually do." Dr. Rous also cautioned that a false-negative PSA exists at about 20 percent of the time in his population study, that is, a normal or low PSA is reported when it should be elevated and prostate cancer is indeed present. You should note too that prostate cancer releases about ten times more PSA in the blood than BPH per gram of tissue. Prostatitis, unlike BPH, is known to significantly increase PSA levels that look suspiciously like prostate cancer.

The PSA is a large molecule and is normally passed from epithelial and cancerous cells of the prostate gland into the small blood vessels or capillaries. The reason why there is a higher escape of PSA from prostate cancer tissues or tumours into the blood rather than from BPH tissues is that basement membranes of prostate cancer cells break down and PSA readily escapes. This disruption of the basement membrane does not readily occur in benign growth such as BPH. An elevated PSA does not automatically confirm that you have cancer, only that there is an abnormal condition within the prostate and a need to further evaluate the condition. Urologist Catalona and many in the medical profession caution that a man with an elevated PSA or when the doubling of the PSA becomes suspicious after 6 months to a year needs to be further investigated with a biopsy. At the end of this chapter a consideration of PSA values and recommendations for a biopsy are presented as guidelines. There is still an ongoing controversy regarding the total PSA or cutoff values and recommendations for a biopsy by some of the outstanding urologists and oncologists in the United States and Canada.

Generally a man who is less than 50 years of age would have a PSA value that could range from 0.2 ug/l to 2.5 ug/l. Between the ages of 50 and 59 years his PSA may range from 2.6 ug/l to 3.5 ug/l; between the ages of 60 to 69 years his PSA may range from 3.6 to 4.5 ug/l, and for a man between 70 and 79 years of age his PSA may range from 4.6 ug/l to 6.5 ug/l or could even be higher or lower according to the book, *Prostate Cancer,* co-authored by urologist Peter Scardino. Do not be surprised if your PSA reading has a low sensitivity of 0.2 ug/l or higher than 4 ug/l if you are between 50 and 60 years of age. Urologist Martin Gleave at the Vancouver Prostate Centre reported that "among males between the ages of 50 and 70 years, about 2 percent of them would have a PSA reading greater than 10 ug/l. Eight percent of them would have a PSA reading between 4 ug/l and 10 ug/l, and 90 percent of this population would have a PSA reading lower than 4 ug/l." Dr. Carter in a *JAMA* article added: "Recognizing that 70 percent of a screened population between 50 and 70 years of age have PSA levels less than 2.0 ng/ml, elimination of annual PSA testing for these men would result in large health care cost savings." What can the PSA tell us about the probability of having cancer? A 2005 report from the *American Cancer Society* stated: "If your level of PSA is in the borderline range between 4 and 10, you have about a 25% chance of having prostate cancer. If it is more than 10, your chance of having prostate cancer is over 67% and increases as your PSA level increases." This information is of immense importance to men who take the PSA test.

During my annual physical examination my doctor performed a DRE. A suspicious lump was discovered by DRE at the age of 57 years; a follow-up PSA reading was only 0.2 ug/l and it should have been elevated - a definite *false negative* reading! PSA alone could not detect my tumour or cancer. To repeat, and it is important to heed this information that Dr. Thompson and co-workers reported in the *New England Journal of Medicine,* it is not surprising to have prostate cancer with a PSA level of 0.5 ng/ml or less. Dr. Catalona also pointed out that small tumours do not cause the PSA to elevate. My tumour was small and confined to the right lateral lobe of my prostate. My doctor referred me to an urologist even though my PSA reading was 0.2 ug/l because he realized that the suspicious lump needed further evaluation. Twelve years following surgery my PSA is less than 0.04 ug/l using the Immulite 2000 assay. I thank my general practitioner whom I have been seeing for the past 25 years for his continued guidance and professionalism.

In general, if the PSA reading is greater than 4 ug/l and DRE is not suspicious for prostate cancer, there is about a 20 percent probability of cancer being present. Dr. Catalona reported that "more than two-thirds of men with PSA levels higher than 10 ug/l are found to have cancer, and in more than half of these cases cancers have spread... The use of PSA measurements in conjunction with rectal examination detects 30-40 percent more cancers than rectal examination alone." If the *DRE screening alone* is performed, about one-third of the cancer would not be detected according to Dr. Gerald Andriole. The findings from the research in England previously cited by Dr. Philip also reported that in patients with normal DRE about one-third had positive biopsies for prostate cancer. However, both the DRE and PSA are regarded as complementary tests to detect prostate cancer.

A biopsy is highly recommended if the PSA level is elevated and a DRE detects a lump or abnormal swelling on the prostate. When an individual takes the PSA test the reading may come back as unusually high and the patient might think cancer is present. The following conditions will collectively elevate a man's PSA and you should be aware of these developments: BPH, prostatitis, urinary tract infections, immediately after a prostate biopsy procedure, soon after having a DRE, several hours after an ejaculation, and after having bladder surgery. Once again, it is *not unusual* for a man to have a PSA value of more than 10 ug/l and not have any malignancy. Men older than 70 years of age would also have higher PSA readings even when no disease is present – aging increases the volume of the prostate as a normal developmental process and the PSA value would be somewhat elevated due to the presence of BPH. Dr. Oesterling noted that the age-specific reference has the potential to make the serum PSA a more discriminating tumour marker for detecting clinically significant cancers in older men as well as potentially curable cancers in younger men.

Dr. Sheldon Marks, in his book on *Prostate & Cancer*, suggested that "the use of tobacco products may inhibit changes in the PSA in spite of the presence of cancer." Smokers beware! The research in the literature reveals that patients who are taking Proscar or finasteride for BPH will have lower PSA values. The following is an interesting piece of information on the use of finasteride. The *National Cancer Institute* in the U.S. conducted a study with Proscar or finasteride to determine the progression of prostate cancer with men in experimental and control groups (placebo). The placebo controlled study of about 19 000 men age 55 and older who took 5 milligrams of finasteride daily. The results were mixed: prostate cancer was detected in 18 percent of the men taking finasteride and in 24 percent in the placebo group but tumours were of a higher grade with the men taking finasteride than in the placebo group. A report of another controlled study with finasteride on 3 040 men found that the men in the finasteride group had a slightly higher rate of positive biopsies than men in the placebo or control group, according to the research by Dr. Patrick Walsh. One wonders about the wisdom of conducting trials using finasteride to determine the extent of prostate cancer or in cancer prevention. Finasteride also masks the PSA level and while it appears low it may give the impression that cancer is not present. In fact, finasteride or dutasteride can cause a reduction in PSA level by about 50 percent.

Will riding a bicycle, motorbike or a horse before taking a PSA test increase the levels? Dr. Tariel and others investigated 133 cyclists of a mean age of 54 years in the Paris to Nice race by having a PSA test done before and after the race. They found that the practice of cycling actually reduced the total PSA. The doctor may also advise the patient to have his PSA test done at a Cancer Clinic a few months following surgery or radiation for more sensitive reading although provincial laboratories report PSA values to sensitivities of less than 0.04 ug/l using the Immulite 2000 assay. A man may wish to have the free PSA test done at the Cancer Clinic laboratory in addition to the total PSA test. A score of zero for the PSA is never reported. A third-generation Immulite PSA assay claims a detection limit of 0.003 ug/l and a functional sensitivity of 0.01 ug/l. The third-generation PSA assay may be beneficial in post-operative cancer progression or from any suspected recurrence.

Studies have shown that the PSA and DRE do not always detect the same tumours. Palpable tumours may be found by DRE but microscopic tumours cannot be detected. A doctor performing a DRE may also miss some tumours, so a PSA may detect tumours that the DRE may have missed. Since prostate cancer can be multifocal, PSA may detect those cancers that the DRE misses. Tumours in the transition zone is rarely detected by DRE but generally by having a biopsy – as mentioned earlier, about 20 percent of prostate cancer arises in the transition zone. Trans-rectal ultrasound may not be able to identify tumours in the transition zone. A PSA test may be used to identify multifocal cancer and any tumours in the transition zone. As mentioned, both the PSA and DRE are used as the optimum procedure for detecting prostate cancer. To get another picture of how PSA values affect cancer progression, one study conducted at Johns Hopkins University found the mean PSA value for organ-confined disease was 5.6; for capsular penetration the PSA value was 7.7. As the cancer became more aggressive and moved into the seminal vesicles, the PSA value rose to 23, and for lymph node involvement in the same study, the PSA was elevated to 26. Of course, not every study conducted will provide similar results as indicated above but it is clear that as the PSA value becomes elevated the cancer has a tendency to spread or metastasize and become more aggressive and it also has the tendency to escape the prostate capsule. PSA values correlate with both prostate size and volume; however, the PSA values correlate more strongly with tumour volume than prostate size in patients.

What are the Recommended PSA Cutoffs?

Dr. Walsh reported that raising the PSA bar over 4.0 as a rule for anyone is not recommended for a biopsy and said "we now recommend a cutoff of 2.5 for men in their forties, a maximum of 3.5 for men in their fifties, and a cutoff of 4 for all other men." Some believe that the cutoff concept may not work in all situations. Urologist Thompson in his investigation of 18 882 men age 55 and older in a Prostate Cancer Prevention Trial stated that "there is no clearly defined PSA cutpoint at which to recommend a biopsy but rather a continuum of prostate cancer risk at all values of PSA." In an article in the New England of Medicine, Dr. Punglia and colleagues pointed out that "if the threshold PSA value for undergoing a biopsy were set at 4.1 ng per milliliter, 85 percent of cancers in younger men and 65 percent in older men would be missed." They went on to say that the "threshold level at which a biopsy is to be recommended should be 2.6 ng/ml, at least in men under 60 years of age, may be reasonable."

In that large study conducted by Dr. Thompson and colleagues, they reported that "biopsy-detected prostate cancer, including high-grade cancers, is not rare among men with PSA levels of 4 ng/ml or less – levels thought to be in the normal range." Though stated earlier, it should be re-emphasized that it is not uncommon for men with a normal PSA levels to develop prostate cancer underscores and there is a need to consider fundamental changes in the approach to diagnosing prostate cancer. One recommendation made some years ago by Urologist Gleave and associates was that "men with a PSA of less than 1.0 and a normal DRE should be re-evaluated every three to four years. Those with a PSA level between 1.0 and 4.0 should be rechecked one year later." Dr. Pickles stated that if a man's PSA is less than 1.0 ng/ml. he should be checked every 5 years. Dr. Hugosson and colleagues in Sweden in their study of 9 972 men between the age of 50 and 65 years with an initial PSA of less than 2, said that they should be rechecked after two years.

The Velocity of PSA and Doubling Time

Your doctor should be aware of any changes in your PSA levels and explain what those changes could imply. Is your PSA rising gradually or not at all or is it doubling every 6 to 10 months? If your PSA was 1.0 last year and one year later it has risen to 1.8, there is some cause for concern. If a man has a smaller prostate gland and his PSA doubling time (PSADT) is within one year, he is of greater risk than a man with a larger prostate gland. The PSADT for early prostate cancer (at stages A or B or T1 to T2) may be about every two years or even longer. If the doubling time is less than 10 months, there is a high probability of metastatic disease according to a Prostate Cancer Research Institute report. In asymptomatic men, Dr. Strum stated that if the PSADT is less than 12 years there is a high probability that cancer is present. The PSADT may be more appropriate in measuring cancer growth than the PSA velocity; following postoperative biochemical failure, shorter PSADT is associated with higher risk of clinical progression. Dr. D'Amico and colleagues evaluated whether men are at risk from prostate cancer after radical prostatectomy. They studied 1 095 men with localized prostate cancer and assessed the rise in PSA, its velocity during the year before diagnosis together with the PSA at diagnosis, including the Gleason score and clinical stage. A PSA velocity of higher than 2.0 ng/ml per year was associated with a high risk of death from prostate cancer despite having had radical prostatectomy.

Other considerations such as a Gleason score and the time from having had surgery or radiation to any biochemical recurrence are clinical parameters that can help patients and physicians make decisions about any additional treatment. Changes in PSA levels are good guidelines in detecting prostate cancers or recurrence. The appropriate cutoff recommended for a biopsy, as suggested by Dr. Catalona, is if the PSA velocity within one year is 0.75 ng/ml. In a report from a 10-year screening study of 26 000 men, a PSA velocity of 0.5 ng/ml within one year was significant enough to recommend a biopsy. Measuring the PSA velocity requires more than one test during the year for more accurate calculations of the rate of increase. From the research cited, a PSA velocity of 0.5 to 0.75 ug/l in one year should be an appropriate benchmark for a biopsy for all men.

Cancerous cells seem to secrete about ten times more PSA than BPH and it is one way to differentiate between benign and cancerous tumours. A doubling time of PSA of less than four to six months should be regarded as significant and a reason to see your urologist or oncologist. Each individual is different and if his PSADT is insignificant within one year, it does not mean that he is cancer free. An ultrasensitive PSA assay should be recommended for checking any recurrent disease since the Immulite 2000 PSA assay takes a longer time to show any significant rise in PSA. By using the ultrasensitive PSA test "31 patients (30%) who were considered in remission by the regular PSA test would be reclassified as having biochemical recurrence" according to Dr. McDermed in an *Insights Newsletter.* The Memorial Sloan-Kettering website provides useful information in predicting disease progression including the PSA velocity for any available data. It is advisable to access that nomogram at: www.mskcc.org/mskcc/html/10088.cfm. Other nomograms discussed in the next chapter are useful predictors of disease progression.

The **density** of the prostate is also an important consideration for the presence of prostate cancer. For the density, the urologist determines the size of the prostate with transrectal ultrasound and divides the PSA number by the prostate volume for its density. For example, if your PSA is 6 and your prostate weighs 40 grams as an estimate from its size, then your prostate density is 0.15. The higher the density the more PSA per cubic centimetre is present and it may signify the presence of cancer. The density is not included in detecting prostate cancer since the PSA velocity and PSADT are more meaningful diagnostic tools.

Total PSA, Free PSA, pro-PSA and uPM3 as Tumour Markers

Researchers are investigating more reliable tumour markers to predict the presence of prostate cancer in addition to the total PSA that is commonly in use. So far the total PSA values in evaluating a man's chances of having prostate cancer and disease progression are considered. Other PSA tests are currently being used and have proven valuable to detect prostate cancer or to determine whether a biopsy is necessary. **Serum PSA** comes in various forms, notably, the **bound, free and pro-PSA** isoforms. The PSA molecule circulating in the blood is bound or attached to other proteins. Bound PSA means that a protein such as alpha-1-antichymotrypsin or alpha-macroglobulin is tagged on to it – it is also referred to as the **complex PSA.** Oftentimes the bound protein is broken off and the PSA becomes free within the prostate gland and bloodstream. When a *total PSA* is taken for most tests, it includes both the free and bound types. By separating the bound and free PSA, it makes the PSA tests more specific, and may indicate how aggressive a cancer is behaving. Thus the free PSA test provides more information to the pathologist or clinician about a man's prostate condition. It is important to know that when a man's PSA elevates because of BPH, more of the PSA is present in the free form. Thus, the **higher** the percent **free PSA** the more likely a man is free of prostate cancer – a higher percent free PSA possibly means good news to the patient or no cancer is likely present, but having a lower free PSA percent could spell bad news. The free PSA in serum has been shown to enhance the specificity of PSA testing for prostate cancer detection.

Prostate cancer is therefore more likely to be present if the ratio of free PSA to total PSA (multiplied by 100) is less than 15 percent. One study done on men with PSA values between 4 and 10 and in conjunction with the free PSA, the investigators were able to diagnose 95 percent of cancers. This is a very high probability rate with a consideration of the free PSA test to determine if a biopsy is needed. In the book *A Guide to Surviving Prostate Cancer*, Dr. Walsh writes: "If the free PSA is less than

15 percent, it's more likely that all of the PSA is coming from cancer, that the cancer is significant in size, and that it will prove aggressive." The *American Cancer Society* in 2005 was more cautious in their findings and concluded that "if your PSA is of a borderline range of 4 to 10 ng/ml, a low percent-free PSA of less than 10% it means that your likelihood of having prostate cancer is about 50% and that you should have a biopsy..." Dr. Etzioni and investigators analyzed the total and free PSA from blood stored from cancer patients and controls. They noted that combining the total and free PSA showed modest improvements over the total PSA. However, they found that by using the percent free PSA below a threshold of 4ng/ml of total PSA could translate into a reduction of unnecessary biopsies. There is the potential of avoiding any unnecessary biopsy when the result from a free PSA test is known.

A *Multicenter Clinical Trial* was conducted and included 379 men with prostate cancer and 394 men with BPH, with all men having total PSA values ranging from 4.0 to 10.0 ng/ml. That study, conducted by Dr. Catalona and co-workers, reported that when the free PSA was less than 10 percent, prostate cancer risk increased to over 56 percent; if a free PSA ranged from 15-20 percent the probability of having prostate cancer was 20 percent, and for a free PSA of 20-25 percent the probability of having cancer was reduced to 16 percent. If the free PSA was greater than 25 percent, the risk of prostate cancer was greatly reduced to 8 percent. The cancers associated with greater than 25 percent free PSA were more prevalent in older patients with BPH and the cancers were less threatening. For a biopsy, Dr. Catalona and colleagues suggest "a cutoff of less than 25 percent or less of free PSA is recommended for patients in conjunction with a total PSA between 4 and 10 ng/ml and a palpable *benign* gland, regardless of patient age or prostate size." Ask your doctor about getting the free blood serum PSA test done in addition to the total PSA. If your PSA velocity looks suspicious you should also ask for a free PSA test in conjunction with the total PSA.

Serum **pro-PSA** consists of several molecular forms of the free PSA and one form of the pro-PSA is believed to have significant advantage over the total or free PSA from one study. One type of pro-PSA is elevated in prostate cancers and identifies the more aggressive forms of prostate cancer; it could distinguish between cancer and benign conditions in men when the total PSA is from 2.5 to 10 ng/ml. In a study reported by Dr.

Catalona and colleagues in *The Journal of Urology* using 1 091 serum specimens with 555 specimens of PSA ranging from 2 to 4 ng/ml, and 536 specimens of PSA ranging from 4 to 10 ng/ml, "the percent pro-PSA was superior to percent free and calculated complexed PSA for the detection of prostate cancer in the (total) PSA range of 2 to 10 ng/ml." Furthermore, the pro-PSA detected more aggressive cancers from Gleason score of 7 or greater and/or extra-capsular tumour extension. In men with greater than 25 percent free PSA, or men who would not be recommended for a biopsy, the percent pro-PSA may be able to detect most cancers while avoiding two-thirds of unnecessary biopsies. Pro-PSA biochemical markers could eliminate unnecessary biopsies because of its accuracy in detecting prostate cancer and higher grade tumours over the total and free PSA. The pro-PSA seems to be a more specific marker than the total PSA or free PSA but at the time of writing the pro-PSA test was not available for the general population. Dr. Lein and other investigators studied the use of the pro-PSA in a Multicenter Clinical Trial of 2 055 white men. Their study showed "no improvement in diagnostic accuracy when comparing the pro-PSA and the ratios with total PSA or total to free PSA." Researchers contend that further studies should focus on the determination of a single pro-PSA rather than on the combined forms of pro-PSA.

You will recall in Chapter 2 the mention of a new prostate cancer genetic-urine marker, **uPM3**, that was investigated as a possible tumour marker for prostate cancer. That test is now available as the first urine-based genetic marker for prostate cancer, and the gene identified is referred to as PCA3. The uPM3 test was reported in *PCRI Insights Newsletter* in May 2005 and in Urology in 2004; it is now produced by Bostwick Laboratories and available in the United States. "The uPM3 test predicts cancer as confirmed by prostate biopsy with 81 % accuracy, compared to 47 % accuracy with the PSA" according to oncologist Strum in *Insights*. Urologist Partin said that "the uPM3 test is an exciting new urine test to help men make critical decisions regarding early detection for prostate cancer." Incidentally, the uPM3 tumour marker at time of writing was trading in the Toronto Stock Market and managed by DiagnoCure in Quebec. Doctors should continue to recommend the total and free PSA tests to monitor a man's prostate condition until the uPM3 test and pro-PSA test become more widely available; more research is required on the reliability of the latter two tests before they are offered to the public. Dr. Xiaoju Wang and other investigators reported that *autoantibodies* against peptides (segments of proteins) derived from prostate cancer tissue had performed better than PSA in identifying prostate cancer and could be used as a screening test. In the *Cancer Research journal* of May 2005, Dr. Barbara Paul and researchers identified an **early prostate cancer antigen** (EPCA) that was expressed only in prostate cancer individuals; it shows that EPCA has the potential to be a more specific blood marker for prostate cancer than the total PSA. More tests are required with larger populations to confirm the efficacy of EPCA. One novel protein reported by Dr. Nam and colleagues, referred to as total prostate secretory protein of 94 amino acids, produced by the prostate gland requires further study to determine its use as a tumour marker.

Recommendations and Caution

The American Cancer Society and the American Urological Association recommend an annual PSA testing and digital rectal examination at the age of 50 years and beginning at the age of 40 to 45 years for high risk individuals, such as those with a family history of prostate cancer and men of African origin who are at a greater risk of developing prostate cancer. Some years ago the Canadian Urological Association stated: "The DRE and PSA measurements increase the early detection of clinically significant prostate cancer. The DRE and PSA tests are indicated in the investigation of men having prostate cancer and in the management of men with prostate cancer. Until proof of the benefits of early detection is available we recommend that the PSA test not be offered as a screening tool for prostate cancer except in the context of a randomized screening trial. Men considering having these tests should be made aware of the potential benefits and risks."

A 1997 National Prostate Cancer Forum in Canada recommended that "all men should have the opportunity to undergo a PSA...we therefore recommend that men should be made aware of the benefits and risks of early detection testing using PSA and DRE, so they can make informed decisions." In 2005, in *The Journal of Urology,* a study conducted by Dr. Kopek and colleagues in Toronto and funded by the Canadian Cancer Society (CCS), demonstrated that early PSA screening may reduce the risk of metatastic prostate cancer. A CCS representative, Dr. Barbara Whylie, stated that "the study suggests that early PSA screening may reduce the risk of metastatic prostate cancer." Even though the research has not been fully investigated to demonstrate that PSA screening reduces mortality from prostate cancer, PSA screening detects cancer earlier for curative treatment using modern therapies. Early diagnosis is preferable to late diagnosis since there is no cure for advanced prostate cancer. The data over the past 10 years showed a 25 percent decline in mortality rate in Canada of cases diagnosed from prostate cancer during the PSA era. Some opponents to population-based PSA screening argue that the natural history of prostate cancer is not well known; others contend that the tests used for screening may not be effective. The total and free PSA tests have proven to be the best tools available to detect malignancy and will continue to be used until other proven and more reliable tests are established.

General practitioners are also being educated about the usefulness and limitations of the total PSA test; they must be prepared to discuss the advantages and disadvantages of prostate screening with patients. Despite the limitations, the PSA test remains the best detector of prostate cancer tumour. Like women who are concerned about their health and especially with the high incidence of breast cancer, men too are becoming more concerned about prostate cancer in their lives than any other disease. Many men believe that some of the benefits of earlier detection, diagnosis and treatment have resulted in the decline in mortality from prostate cancer. Men at the two Prostate Support Groups I attend swear by the fact that the PSA test has helped in their diagnosis and allowed them to have earlier curable treatment. In a study conducted by Dr. Bader and colleagues in Germany, 1 731 men who underwent radical prostatectomy were evaluated retrospectively for their PSA levels. The study demonstrated that prostate cancer with a PSA of less than or equal to 8 ng/ml did not initially seem to be a harmless cancer but in more than one-third of the patients studied the tumour was not organ confined, and 6 percent even showed regional lymph node metastases. I personally believe that much caution should be used in the interpretation of the total PSA test *by itself.* A total PSA value of greater than 4 ug/l or a PSA velocity of 0.75 ug/l within one year is cause for concern.

Men under the age of 60 years should have a biopsy done for a PSA cutoff at 2.6 ug/l as suggested by some investigators. Dr. Thompson and colleagues, on the other hand, suggested that there should not be any specific cutoff point for the PSA but rather a continuum of prostate cancer risk at all values of PSA. For the present time, both the total PSA and DRE will continue to determine the need to further evaluate a man's prostate condition and to indicate whether a biopsy is necessary. A PSA should be recommended at an earlier age of 40 to 45 years for men who are at risk. There is some cause for concern, especially if there is a family history of prostate cancer or if a man is of African descent. Many men seem to be making the right decisions by requesting the PSA test. The Canadian Prostate Cancer Network recommends that men should begin PSA testing yearly at age 40 and an annual DRE. Would having a PSA test cause tens of thousands of men to needlessly worry about their health? A 50 year old man, with the advice of his physician, should consider having a total PSA test done as well as a free PSA test. The cost of the test is usually covered by the health care system.

The Biopsy

What is a biopsy and how is it performed? What are the recommendations for having a biopsy? Reasons to perform a biopsy include the discovery of a lump or a nodule during a DRE and/or if the PSA level is suspiciously elevated. The information provided in this chapter on PSA values, its velocity and doubling time should be included in the decision to have a biopsy by patient consultation with his doctor. Your urologist or oncologist will inform you of what you need to do in preparation for having a biopsy, including which medications to avoid. You may have to take an enema, take the antibiotics recommended to avoid the risk of infection, and be sure not take any blood thinning agents for the last week to ten days before the test. The biopsy procedure is not a complicated one and it takes little time to have it done. An **ultrasound** examination procedure is carried out to determine the size and location of any prostate abnormality before and during the biopsy procedure; the entire prostate gland is scanned by ultrasound. The ultrasound probe is lubricated and inserted into the rectum. The procedure is at first uncomfortable but that feeling soon disappears. Patients are told to relax and not to tense up the muscles in much the same way as when having a DRE. Ultrasound is a way of getting a picture of tissues by bouncing sound waves off the area to be examined. The biopsy needle is guided into the prostate by ultrasound, and tissue samples or cores are extracted from any suspected tumours and from other zones by suction. The biopsy procedure sounds like a horrifying experience but my urologist pleasantly surprised me and I experienced little discomfort. I was expecting to experience a great deal of pain and was quite concerned about the procedure when I had first heard about it.

A spring-loaded, hand-held biopsy gun (and this sounds like a shooting machine but is not) is used by the urologist. To put you at ease, you should not be too concerned by being subjected to this procedure. The urologist may also feel for the presence of any tumour while guiding the needle; more often the needle is inserted alongside the ultrasound probe. There is often a tinge of blood present in the urine or ejaculate following a biopsy but that should disappear in a few days. It is advisable to abstain from sexual intercourse until the bleeding has stopped. Your urologist will advise you on activities following the biopsy. When I had my biopsy done my only concern was being subjected to that humiliating position, and I thought for a moment of the many women who are routinely subjected in the same manner for their regular pelvic examinations. Before my procedure began an attending female nurse recognized me as her former biology teacher and we had a good laugh about that unusual and unique reunion. In small talk, my urologist then made a comment that he did not study high school biology courses and I wondered if that earlier lack of the rat anatomy would affect my impending surgery!

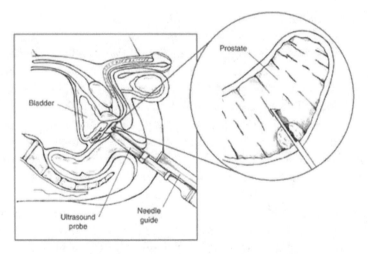

Figure 5.2: Transrectal ultrasound and prostate biopsy using suction needle. Adapted from the National Kidney and Urologic Diseases Information Clearinghouse, National Institute of Health.

The biopsy procedure went well and was efficiently performed. I began to regain the confidence in my urologist's ability to locate my prostate gland and his knowledge of anatomy; in my opinion, he is an excellent surgeon as we will learn later about my radical prostatectomy or surgical procedure. The popping sound of the biopsy gun as the needle is passed through the rectal wall into the prostate gland to extract the samples was more terrifying than the actual needle penetration. When my urologist collected the tissue samples I asked to see them and wanted to know about the histological procedure since I felt that it may be useful to me as a biology teacher, not knowing that one or more samples would later prove to be cancerous. From 6 to 9 core samples from a biopsy may be taken to establish the extent of cancer as well as the grade and stage of any malignancy. Within minutes after the biopsy I was in my car and on my way home. It takes one to two weeks to get the results from the pathology lab. One should avoid putting any pressure on the prostate so avoid riding a bicycle, motor bike or a horse after the biopsy. I called my doctor's office for an appointment to see him following the biopsy and I was bracing for the worst news. My doctor was earlier trying to contact me but I was out of town. As it turned out, my prostate cancer cells proved positive for malignancy but I will discuss that topic in detail later.

One warning, a negative biopsy does not prove that you do not have cancer but your chances of having cancer are quite low. If the first biopsy carried out misses any suspected cancer and the report is negative, but if your PSA had been suspiciously high and/or if DRE has been done and identified a lump in the prostate, another biopsy should be carried out in a few months. There is the possibility of the biopsy needle missing a small tumour or section of the gland. Also, many cancers are multifocal or found in several sites within the gland and the biopsy suction needle may not catch them. Insist on having six or more different biopsy needle samples from your prostate gland. An interesting point to note is that the Gleason grade on initial needle biopsy is an inexact predictor of the final grade following radical prostatectomy. The Gleason grade and scores are explained in the next chapter. A Gleason score following radical prostatectomy from the pathology findings is a more accurate indicator of patient prognosis than before treatment. "Patients with biopsy Gleason score of 6 who are under-graded are at significantly higher risk for adverse pathological features and biochemical recurrence than patients who remain with Gleason score of 6 or less on final pathology findings" according to Dr. Paul Sved and colleagues in *The Journal of Urology.* Dr. Dan Vick, a pathologist, noted that between 13 and 36 percent of post-surgical Gleason scores are elevated compared to the score made at the time of initial biopsy. The procedure by Dr. Vick is to produce 4 slides for each biopsy core and it takes about 45 minutes to evaluate a single case of 6 biopsy cores. A twelve-year study conducted by Dr. Bektic and colleagues in Austria found that taking 15 biopsy cores improved the concordance between initial biopsy and prostatectomy Gleason score than by having fewer needle biopsies. The Gleason score, its grade and implications are discussed in Chapter 6.

Further Procedures to Assess the Prostate Condition

One should note that transrectal ultrasound is not 100% accurate and it may miss a malignant lesion, warns urologist Larry Goldenberg. The transition zone, the region closest to the prostatic urethra, may not reveal any tumour by ultrasound when indeed one may be present. "The peripheral zone is the origin of 75% of prostatic adenocarcinomas ... about 25% of prostate cancers arise in either the transition zone or the central zone," according to Dr. Gleave and others. One should note too that the entire exterior of the prostate is not palpable through DRE; the entire front lobe is not palpable and some tumours may even be missed by DRE. A newer technique being used, known as *colour Doppler ultrasound,* measures blood flow within the prostate and has an advantage over the conventional black and white imaging ultrasound. Dr. Frauscher found that colour Doppler targeted-biopsy detected as many cancers as systematic biopsy with fewer than half the number of cores; using the colour enhanced targeted-biopsy alone is a "reasonable approach for decreasing the number of biopsy cores." Because tumours often have more blood vessels surrounding them, the Doppler ultrasound procedure also makes the biopsy more accurate.

Other sophisticated tests, but seldom carried out, may include a lymphangiogram; it is an X-ray that makes use of a special dye to determine whether the cancer has spread to the lymph nodes. A new technique to identify lymph node metastasis was investigated by Dr. Harisinghani and colleagues. They tested whether highly lymphotropic superparamagnetic nanoparticles which enter the lymph nodes could be used in conjunction with MRI to detect nodal metastases. Eighty patients who underwent lymph-node resection or biopsy were investigated. The findings revealed

"the detection of small and otherwise undetectable lymph-node metastases in patients with prostate cancer." Another test, the *CAT scan* using a
series of X-rays provides several views of the pelvic regions and lymph
nodes but that test may not be effective in determining if cancer is present. The experimental use of a *monoclonal antibody* attached to a radioactive isotope appears to identify some but not all sites of prostate cancer
outside the prostate gland. A new form of monoclonal antibody developed
by Cornell College of Medicine appears to detect small amounts of
prostate cancer as an additional tool for detecting extracapsular cancer. In
Chapter 9, under If Prostate Cancer Returns, the use of the ProstaScint
imaging seems to detect more lymph node cancer by using more refined
techniques. *Nomograms* are also used to predict lymph node involvement
as well as seminal vesicles invasion as discussed in the next chapter.
Cystoscopy is a procedure which uses a light source the tube (Figure 5.3)
is inserted into the opening of the penis and the urethra.

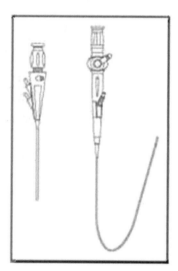

Figure 5.3: A rigid and flexible cystoscope. Adapted from the National Cancer
Institute Visuals.

The cystoscopic procedure is uncomfortable but becomes less painful
as a local anesthetic gel is applied into the urethra during the procedure.
Cystoscopy is used to determine the size of the urethral diameter, prostate
or bladder condition but the procedure is *not* performed to detect prostate
cancer. In future the combination of MRI with newer tests such as the

lymphotropic superparamagnetic nanoparticles may become scanning tools to assess the stage of prostate and other cancers.

Summary Recommendations

If you are a young healthy male in your twenties and thirties and have no prostate problems, the PSA test is not recommended for you. Healthy men in their forties with no familial risk should decide for themselves (and with guidance from physicians) whether to have a PSA test or be satisfied with only having a DRE performed during a physical examination. As stated previously, DRE may miss malignant tumours and it is not completely effective in detecting cancer. Age, any prostate symptoms and familial risk are factors that should be considered when requesting a PSA test. Dr. Patrick Walsh, the pioneer of the nerve-sparing technique, and colleagues at Johns Hopkins University, recommend that you should have a biopsy if your DRE detects a tumour even when your PSA is as low as 0.2 ug/l. If your DRE is negative, the next step depends on your PSA value and age for a possible biopsy.

Dr. Walsh recommends that you should have a biopsy when the DRE is negative but if your PSA values are:

- Greater than 2.5 and you are between forty to forty nine years of age.

- Greater than 3.5 and you are between fifty to fifty nine years of age.

- Greater than 4 and you are sixty years or older.

- Lower than the above PSA ranges but the PSA has increased by more than 1.5 over the last two years.

The above PSA cutoff values are mere guidelines and that specific PSA cutoffs may not be the answer to indicate when a biopsy is to be recommended. With the advent of the PSA and its widespread medical use in the 1990s and since, by checking your serum PSA and understanding how it behaves over several months and years, that is, its velocity and doubling time, you could predict the recommended course of action. It seems to make sense to have your cancer detected earlier for a curative treatment. The combination of PSA values, PSA velocity or doubling time, DRE, clinical staging, Gleason score and grade contribute significantly to the prediction of the pathological stage of localized prostate cancer as well as any extracapsular cancer.

Not everyone seems to agree that regular screening with PSA and DRE is the best path to follow. Urologist Goldenberg puts it succinctly as follows: "Early detection is really essential. A 60 year old man dying of prostate cancer used to be a 50 year old man who had curable prostate cancer." The long-term natural history of untreated early stage prostate cancer was examined by Dr. Johansson and others. They concluded that most prostate cancers diagnosed at an early stage have an indolent (tiny cancer with no immediate threat to life) course of tumour progression, but in the long term aggressive metastatic disease may develop. The investigation by Dr. Johansson supports the use of early radical treatment among patients with an estimated life expectancy exceeding 15 years.

By lowering the PSA threshold from 4.0 to 2.6 in men under the age of 60 years, the number of prostate cancers detected would increase. Why wait until the PSA rises to 4.0 when a worse case scenario may likely develop? With a PSA of 4.0 "in 30% of the men (having radical prostatectomy) the cancer had extended to the edge of the prostate or beyond" warns Dr. Catalona. Drs. Punglia and Catalona published an article in the *New England Journal of Medicine* and recommended lowering of the PSA threshold from 4.0 to 2.6. Urologist's Walsh's age-PSA relationships as presented above could still be valid considerations for patients and physicians. Drs. Punglia and Catalona concluded that with a PSA benchmark set at 4.1 ng/ml "85% of cancers in young men and 65% in older men would be missed." Dr. Thompson and others found that high grade cancers are not uncommon among men with a PSA of 4.0 or less. The patient therefore should seriously consider having a biopsy regardless of age if his PSA is 2.6 ug/l or higher. In a *JAMA* article in 2005, Dr. Thompson and colleagues stated that lowering the PSA threshold "will increase biologically inconsequential cancers...and there is no clearly defined PSA cut point at which to recommend a biopsy."

One is left somewhat confused about the reliability of the **total** PSA test and threshold levels for having a biopsy. The free PSA test should be added to make the diagnosis more meaningful and it should become more widely available to patients in Canada. Patients indeed become confused about the reliability and validity of PSA testing and generally have to rely on the advice of their primary care physicians. At the time of writing, I

spoke with a few general practitioners who were not aware of the importance of the free PSA test and how it was interpreted. So what should the
patient do if his general practitioner has not been fully informed about the
different PSA tests? What should the patient know about PSA tests and his
chances of having prostate cancer?

With a negative DRE, urologist Scardino summarized the following
information of the probability of finding prostate cancer: for a PSA of 2 –
4 there is a 15 percent probability that cancer is present; for a PSA of 4 –
10, there is a 25 percent chance that cancer is present, and with a PSA of
greater than 10, there is a 50 percent probability that prostate cancer is
present. Urologist Walsh, on the other hand, reported that with a PSA
greater than 10, about 65 percent of men were found to have prostate cancer. My advice to all men who are being tested for prostate problems is to
keep accurate records of past tests and your medical history. Have a
record of your total PSA values, free PSA percent, PSA velocity, and what
has your doctor told you or discovered from a DRE. What are your past
or present symptoms, if any? What was your Gleason grade and the two
Gleason numbers or score if a biopsy was done? Aside from prostate concerns, did your doctor have you take other tests for monitoring the levels
of cholesterol, LDL, HDL, triglyceride or glucose? Have you been
assessed for blood chemistry, liver, kidney, thyroid function and other
functions? When was the last time you had those tests done including others not listed above? Did you have your waist circumference checked
every few months for any increasing signs of obesity? Have you had your
blood pressure checked and when did you last have a complete physical
examination? Be sure to review and monitor any past test results which
you should have on file and to discuss the implications of any test results
when you see your doctor.

Chapter 6

The Staging and Grading
of Prostate Cancer

By reading this chapter you will learn:

- Symptoms of prostate diseases.
- The Tumour Node Metastasis or TNM staging system
  and indications or characteristics in staging of malignancy.
- The progression of prostate cancer in the Whitmore-Jewett
  and TNM staging systems.
- Suggested treatment options for each staging level(s).
- Using mathematical models or nomograms to predict
  the extent of cancer and to assess treatment options.
- What is the Gleason score and grade?
- The importance of the Gleason grade in detecting
  progression of cancer.
- How tests could establish a man's prostate profile.

Symptoms of Prostate Problems

It is worth remembering that there are no early warning signs or symptoms of prostate cancer in most cases. If the cancer is at stages A or B (T1a through to T2c), a man is unlikely to experience any symptoms of cancer; symptoms may not even be experienced at a later staging even after cancer has invaded the seminal vesicles, lymph nodes or in distant metastases. Prostate cancer is generally slow growing and many men will not experience any symptoms before the diagnosis is made. Symptoms are

111

generally experienced when prostate cancer is at an advanced stage. Some of the possible *common symptoms* and abnormalities of prostate problems including prostatitis, benign hyperplasia and prostate cancer:

1. Frequency and difficulty in urinating, especially at night.
2. Leakage of urine into underwear garment.
3. Straining to empty the bladder or inability to urinate.
4. The urgency to urinate.
5. Pain or burning sensation upon urination.
6. Difficulty in starting or stopping the urine flow.
7. Presence of blood in the urine.
8. Continuing back pain in the lower back, pelvis, or upper thighs; bone pain, sudden weight loss of a few kilograms, constant fatigue and weakness generally indicate the presence of advanced prostate cancer.

These symptoms are not solely for prostate cancer. From those symptoms, it is not easy to specify whether they are indications of prostate cancer or of other prostate diseases – many symptoms are shared with other prostate diseases including prostate cancer. Do not needlessly worry if symptoms of prostate conditions develop, think that the worst is at hand or jump to conclusions without further testing. However, number eight on the list above is indicative of advanced prostate cancer. Your doctor will advise you on the plan of action should symptoms develop. Generally, a referral to an urologist will be the appropriate course of action for your general practitioner to take when prostate problems or symptoms are suspicious.

Staging Systems

There are four general stages of the progression of prostate cancer disease. These staging levels are categorized from A to D in the Whitmore-Jewett system that groups patients into distinct categories based on clinical stage, pathological size, and the extent of the tumour as defined by urologists and oncologists. Is the cancer indolent? How big is the tumour? Is it confined? How much of the gland does it occupy? Has the cancer left the prostate capsule. The answers to these important questions determine the stage of cancer. Clinical staging determines the kind of treatment that will follow, based on the results of tests such as the DRE, PSA and a biopsy. Urologists and oncologists generally use the Tumour-Node-Metastasis staging system or TNM that was last revised in 2003, based on the sub-classification of prostate conditions and tumours. The TNM system is used to assess microscopic to macroscopic size of the tumour or tumours, cancer progression or the extent of disease within the prostate gland, or whether seminal vesicles or any lymph node invasion are involved, and the extent of metastases. The summary of the TNM staging provided in this chapter illustrates how cancer unfolds. The progression of disease in the conventional and generalized staging system from A to D will also be included with the comparative staging of the TNM system that is more commonly used by doctors and clinicians.

Summary of the TNM Classification System

Stage	Indications in this Stage
TX	Tumour cannot be assessed
TO	No evidence of primary tumour
T1	Cancer is present but is not palpable or visible by imaging
T1a	Tumour found incidental when BPH is done by TURP; present in 5 percent of tissue and cancer is well differentiated
T1b	Found by TURP for BPH; present in more than 5 percent of tissues; grade may be moderately differentiated or even higher
T1c	Detected by needle biopsy and with elevated PSA
T2	Tumour confined within the prostate; doctor can feel a lump by DRE
T2a	Involving less than half of one lobe of the prostate and palpable
T2b	A larger tumour is present by DRE, involving more than half of one lobe but not both lobes
T2c	The tumour is present on more than one lobe of the prostate; it is spreading within the prostate
T3	Tumour extends through the prostate capsule
T3a	Tumour extends beyond the capsule on one or perhaps both sides – likely involvement of the seminal vesicles
T3b	Bilateral penetration of tumour and involvement of the seminal vesicles
T3c	Progression through seminal vesicles and perhaps beyond

Stage	Indications in this Stage
T4	Involves structures including the bladder neck and or/adjacent tissues; massive tumour is palpable.
T4a	Invades the bladder neck, external sphincter, or rectum
T4b	Extension into muscles of the pelvic region
NO	Cancer has not metastasized into lymph nodes
N1	Single lymph node metastasis
N2	One or more nodes involved; size of 2 cm to 5 cm
N3	Metastasis larger than 5 cm in lymph node
MO	No distant metastasis beyond the pelvic region
M1a	Distant metastasis and distant lymph node involvement
M1b	Cancer has metastasized in the bone
M1c	The cancer has involved other sites such as the liver.

Staging of Prostate Cancer

The summary of the TNM system above was updated from many sources since it was last modified in 2003. Treatment options for all stages are only suggestions as they are presented in the literature. Your doctor and other health care professionals will provide the optimum advice for treatment and you should *not* use the treatment options in this book as medical advice. National Comprehensive Cancer Network provides a good website for treatment guidelines. You can download "Prostate Cancer Treatment Guidelines for Patients" at: www.nccn.org/patient-/_gls/_english/_prostate/contents.asp#.

Stage A or **T1 through to T1c** staging of disease is recognized in about 20 to 25 percent of patients with adenocarcinoma of the prostate, according to an American College of Surgeons survey. This cancer is never detected by the normal digital rectal examination (DRE) because it is not palpable, but is detected co-incidentally by microscopic investigation after transurethral resection of the prostate or TURP. Cancer at this stage is usually detected in men with BPH condition and after a biopsy analysis for suspicious PSA values. A biopsy sample taken from the transition zone of the prostate following TURP procedure reveals malignancy in about one in ten cases. About 20 percent of prostate cancers arise in the transition zone. Stages T1 to T1c include primary minute tumours, confined to one area of the prostate and are generally well differentiated in Gleason grade. In stage A1 or T1 the cancer is clinically not apparent, not palpable or visible by imaging with an ultrasound. Of course many small cancers are multifocal and are usually not found in only one site of the gland.

For most men, well differentiated microscopic malignancy at stage A is the common Gleason grade. An advanced stage A or T1c stage is identified generally when a man's PSA becomes elevated; a needle biopsy then confirms the stage and grade of cancer. Neo-adjuvant hormonal therapy is sometimes recommended before surgery or radiation therapy for cancer at this stage. Brachytherapy, an important treatment option, has been increasing in Canada and has become one alternative treatment option for organ-confined cancer with men having a lower Gleason grade. In my opinion, surgery is often the optimum treatment option if a tumour(s) is confined to the prostate, is well to moderately differentiated in grade, and if the patient is less than 70 years of age, and in good health. The important question is which treatment will best provide an optimum cure. If a man's life expectancy is less than 10 years or he is in poor health and experiencing the latter conditions, then watchful waiting or active surveillance may be considered. In addition, hormone therapy for an older man with a life expectancy of ten years and confined prostate cancer may be considered.

The First Palpable Stage

Stage B or **T2 to T2c** stage of cancer may be detected by DRE. In the main, this stage of cancer is confined to the prostate capsule but you cannot be completely sure. A Stage B1 tumour may measure less than 2 cm in diameter or there may be tiny non-palpable tumours residing in several places within the gland at this stage. The tumour may also be greater than 2 cm in diameter but is still confined to one lobe of the prostate in stages T2 to T2b. If the tumours have advanced onto two lobes, the staging will be advanced to T2c or a B3 stage. "Based on the assumption that all patients without capsular penetration are cured, we estimate treatment efficacy to be 100 percent for well-differentiated tumors; for moderately differentiated tumors treatment efficacy was 72 percent, and 35 percent effective for poorly differentiated tumors," according to an earlier study by Dr. Craig Fleming in the *Journal of the American Medical Association*.

Unfortunately, not all of the so named B sub-stages may be confined to the prostate; under-staging of tumour development has been well documented by many researchers. In an earlier report, urologist John Warner wrote in the B.C. Medical Journal that "experience at Memorial Sloan-Kettering Cancer Center has shown that 64 percent of patients undergoing radical prostatectomy for localized cancer (clinical stage B) had positive surgical margins with tumor extension beyond the prostate capsule or into the seminal vesicle." It is sometimes difficult to assess the precise staging of a man's cancer and it is not uncommon to have under-staging of prostate cancer. A biopsy is one way to determine the grade of the cancer and the possible extent of the cancer in the gland by the number of positive biopsies collected. Under-staging is not uncommon even when the PSA is less than 4 ug/l. If the PSA is higher than 10 ug/l, about 65 percent of the time cancer will be present but its extent in the prostate gland cannot be determined by PSA values only. As the PSA elevates the tumour volume increases and the greater is the probability of extra capsular penetration. With an abnormal DRE and PSA level of greater than 10 ug/l, there is a high probability that prostate cancer is present and it is likely to spread. Experience at Johns Hopkins in one study reported by urologist Walsh, indicated that with a PSA of over 7, capsular penetration was noted; a PSA of over 20 generally involves cancer in the seminal vesicles and lymph nodes.

The urologist or oncologist may suggest alternative treatment options depending on the age of the patient and the extent of his cancer for stage B. If prostate cancer cells are poorly differentiated, that is, the cancer has spread or is at increased risk of doing so within the prostate, together with a reported elevated PSA, treatment could be by external beam radiation in the pelvic region rather than by opting for surgery. However, if surgery is performed on such a patient and later found to have recurrence of disease from a rising PSA, then salvage radiotherapy would be a recommended option. Hormonal therapy may also be used before, during and following surgery or radiation. Dr. Gleave and colleagues noted that eight months of neoadjuvant hormone therapy before radical prostatectomy resulted in low positive margin rates and reduced PSA levels. The standard treatment options for stages T1 through to T2c staging (A and B) are multifold depending on the patient's health condition, age, tumour volume, the number of positive biopsy cores, PSA and Gleason grade and score. Options for treatment of prostate cancer at stage B, depending on your profile, may include one or more of the following treatments: external beam radiation therapy, brachytherapy, radical prostatectomy, hormonal therapy or active surveillance. Alternative treatment options such as high intensity focused ultrasound (HIFU) or cryotherapy is also available for patients with confined prostate cancer and especially for those men who do not want surgery or radiation. Patients and physicians should investigate the latter two treatment options carefully before deciding on whether to proceed with either HIFU or cryosurgery. At the time of writing, HIFU was not approved in the U.S. but is widely used in Britain, France and Germany. HIFU is being offered in Toronto. A younger patient who is in good health will generally be advised to have surgery, especially for a well or moderately differentiated tumour(s) and one that is believed to be confined to the prostate. For an older patient with confined prostate tumour and experiencing other health problems, watchful waiting or active surveillance could be his option. However, external beam radiation and/or brachytherapy with adjuvant hormonal therapy for intermediate to high risk patients may be the recommended treatment options. If surgery is the recommended option, the urologist sometimes puts the patient on a neo-adjuvant hormone therapy in order to downsize the prostate volume. The decision for opting for any particular treatment is made by the patient and his physician(s) when his profile is known and assessed.

In a survey conducted by Dr. Pound and colleagues on men who had surgery between 1982 and 1997 by a single surgeon for clinically localized prostate cancer without neo-adjuvant therapy, 82 percent remained disease free after 15 years. However, do not conclude that men of all ages should rush to have surgery performed as the only option available. According to Dr. Catalona, in uncontrolled studies, "the 15-year survival rates among patients with clinically localized disease who were treated with radical prostatectomy were excellent: 86 to 93 percent." The National Institutes of Health in one study concluded that the 10-year survival rates for radical prostatectomy and radiation therapy were similar. Radiation therapy performed in older patients with advanced tumours for localized disease experienced a "15-year rate of disease-free survival of 45 to 85 percent" according to Dr. Catalona in an article in a *New England Journal of Medicine* article. Details of all known treatment options for prostate cancer appear in Chapters 7 and 9.

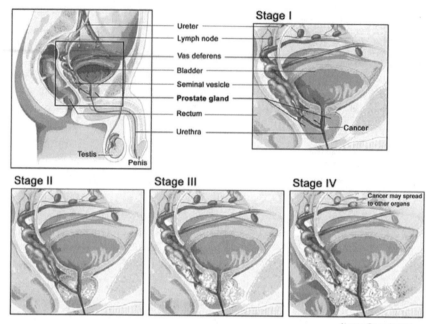

Figure 6.1: Stages I – IV outline changes within the prostate. Stage 1 (possibly T1b - T1c) is a small tumour. Stage II (T2c) shows bilateral growth of tumour and stage III (T3b) represents extra-capsular extension into seminal vesicles. In stage IV (N2+), the cancer involves adjacent tissues, the lymph nodes and other organs. Adapted from the National Cancer Institute Visuals.

Progression of Disease

Stage C or **T3 to T4b** type of prostate cancer has advanced through the capsule of the prostate gland. Extension through the prostate capsule may be from one side or it can be bilateral, that is, progression of the cancer is from two sides of the prostate. This condition may arise from stage T3b through to stage T3c; the cancer may also have invaded the seminal vesicles at these sub-stages. Dr. Goldenberg writes that in many studies "up to 25% of men thought to have disease beyond the prostate gland actually have organ-confined disease." Stages T4a and T4b involve invasion of cancer in adjacent tissues such as the bladder neck and sphincter muscle and this cancer could be classified as being in an early stage D cancer. The oncologist or urologist will determine the extent of a man's cancer from his biopsy to assess the cancer volume, Gleason score and grade. If the cancer volume in the prostate increases above 6 cm, then the chances of seminal vesicle involvement will be high. If the total PSA is greater than 10 ug/l and the free PSA is less than 15 percent, with a Gleason score of 8 – 10 and with 2 to 3 positive needle biopsy, then the cancer may be aggressive and the probability of extra capsular penetration of the cancer will be high.

As a reminder, patients may wish to access the *National Comprehensive Cancer Network* (NCCN) website www.nccn.org for treatment guidelines when the stage and other facts are known about the history of prostate cancer or if there is risk of recurrence. Surgery is not the recommended option if the cancer has spread beyond the prostate cap-sule as in stages T4 and M series as well as at T3 to T3c staging. The NCCN recommends that for men of high risk whose cancer is growing outside the prostate gland but not into adjacent tissues, or with a Gleason score of 8-10 or a PSA greater than 20, hormone therapy for 2-3 years along with external beam radiation will be the appropriate treatment option. The individual may still be unaware of his having any prostate cancer symptoms even when cancer has left the prostate capsule and has moved into adjacent tissues or lymph nodes. It should be noted that as the tumour grows the Gleason score tends to rise due to poorer differentiation of cancer cells. Because aggressive cancer cells are different than normal prostate cells, they make less PSA per gram of tissue than well differenti-ated cells so there is no direct correlation with elevation of PSA levels and with increasing degree of malignancy.

How can the oncologist or urologist determine whether the cancer has escaped the capsule of the prostate gland? How can physicians determine the extent of the cancer within the prostate? Several clues and guiding principles are used to make a judgement call but physicians cannot tell with any certainty if some cancer cells have escaped from the prostate wall. The PSA level (total and free PSA), PSA velocity and/or doubling time, the grade of the tumour, the age of the patient, the volume of the tumour, the number of positive biopsies from the samples collected, and ultrasound imaging are all used to determine the extent and aggressive-ness of the cancer. If the grade of the tumour is poorly differentiated and several positive biopsies have been taken, the prediction is that the tumour volume and cancer size are suspiciously enlarged — it has likely spread across the prostate gland and escaped the capsule. You should note that cancer in the transition zone is very slow to escape the prostate capsule even when the PSA has risen to well over 50 ug/l in some patients. In such a situation cancer is curable by surgery or brachytherapy even though the PSA has escalated well above the expected range. You may recall that in one study conducted at Johns Hopkins University when the PSA value was 7.7, capsule penetration was observed. As the PSA rose to 23, it may signal aggressive prostate cancer and seminal vesicle involvement. The positive biopsy samples from the transition zone are significant in making this determination. A new ProstaScint imaging method is used to check for lymph node and distant metastases; the latter procedure is discussed in Chapter 9 under *If Prostate Cancer Returns.*

Looking Into Nomograms

A useful set of mathematical data, or nomograms, are used to determine disease progression. These are the **Partin Tables,** developed by Dr. Alan Partin and colleagues at Johns Hopkins University and based on information from more than 5 000 men who underwent surgery with Dr. Walsh between 1994 and 2000. It predicts the extent of cancer using different PSA range values, Gleason scores and clinical staging. The *Path Stages* in the Partin Tables for disease progression are identified as organ-confined, capsular penetration, seminal vesicles involvement and lymph node involvement. The Partin Tables, or staging nomograms, are designed to help men and their doctors predict the definitive pathological stage before treatment and to determine the best course of action and a second opinion. There is another similar nomogram table developed by Dr. Perry Narayan and his team from data of hundreds of patients. The two systems, **Partin and Narayan**, may be combined to put more meaning into the prediction of disease progression. On a cautionary note, the tables may tend to over generalize; for example, Partin tables cluster PSA ranges and "suggest that a PSA of 10.1 would have an equal risk that his cancer has spread to the lymph nodes as would a man of a PSA of nearly 20.0" was one criticism by urologist Scardino. On the other hand, Dr. Eskicorapci and colleagues in a Turkish study of 1 043 patients whose clinical and pathological findings were assessed for the reliability of Partin Tables and patients subsequently went on to have surgery; they concluded that Partin Tables have a reasonable predictive value for final pathological features such as organ confined disease, seminal vesicle and lymph node involvement in those Turkish patients. Dr. Ross and investigators at Memorial Sloan-Kettering compared nomograms and urologists' predictions for prostate cancer. From studies conducted, they surprisingly found that nomograms performed above the level of the human expert. The Prostate Cancer Research Institute website below also provides very useful information and the Partin Tables can be accessed at: www.prostate-cancer.org under "Risk Assessment" and by clicking on "PC Tools."

Lymph node examination is one way to confirm if the disease has left the prostate margin. The tissues adjacent to the prostate and seminal vesicles may also be investigated if any extracapsular penetration has occurred. If during radical prostatectomy the lymph nodes are found to be positive for cancer, then the surgery may be aborted and the prostate is left intact. Such a patient could best be treated with external beam radiation and hormone manipulation. However, at Johns Hopkins University, some scientists suggest that men with lymph node cancer may derive some benefit by still undergoing radical prostatectomy. Their findings suggest that men who had positive lymph node metastasis and had surgery lived longer – 56 percent of the men who had surgery were still alive after 10 years compared with 34 percent who did not have any surgery and known to have had lymph node cancer. In my opinion, if surgery is carried out on such a patient then salvage radiotherapy and hormonal therapy should be done. The NCCN recommends that for very high risk patients for cancer that has spread to the lymph nodes then men should receive hormonal therapy for 2-3 years including external beam radiation. The **Bluestein Tables** can also be accessed at the same website above and with data provided, lymph node involvement could be predicted based on clinical staging, Gleason grade (not score), and PSA values. Another mathematical model or nomogram was developed by scientists at Memorial Sloan-Kettering and is similar to the Partin Tables. Anyone wishing more information or have questions with the nomogram may contact Memorial Sloan-Kettering at nomograms@mskcc.org. The Memorial Sloan-Kettering website for accessing the nomograms is: http://mskcc.org/-mskcc/html/10088.cfm. Nomograms are not infallible and are not intended to make decisions for the patient without a physician's recommendation. With known data, a patient and his doctor will be able to suggest the course of action to be taken and predict what would likely happen in the future.

The computerized tools or nomograms are meant for those patients who have not been treated as well as those receiving treatment. For example, before a patient can benefit from a nomogram, he must have had a biopsy, a Gleason grade, his PSA done, and his clinical stage determined. It is worth investigating the Partin Tables and the Sloan-Kettering nomograms with your doctor when all the information or data are taken into consideration. It is akin to doing your homework in preparation for your final exam. Dr. Ross and other urologists "suggest that nomograms do not seem to diminish predictive accuracy and they may be of significant benefit in certain clinical decision making settings." Other nomograms have been extensively developed to predict recurrence after surgery, seminal vesicle invasion, lymph node involvement, probability of metastases after 3D conformal external beam radiation, after brachytherapy, and to determine the presence of small, moderately differentiated confined tumours. Dr. Tisman has summarized eight different nomograms for the latter conditions from the research in the article on "Using Nomograms to Predict Pathological Stages and Treatment Outcomes for Patients with Prostate Cancer" that appeared in PCRI Insights, November 2005. Dr. Tisman commented that in the course of his oncology practice, he has been made to feel like "a referee between the urological surgeon and the radiation therapist as they vie for center stage in the treatment of the prostate cancer patient." Indeed each specialist has his or her bias for optimum treatment of patients that may, unfortunately, pose some confusion for the patient who gets caught in the middle. The eight nomograms cited and presented in the article by Dr. Tisman "have been shown to exceed the expertise of physician professional opinion, and often based on physician bias and less than objective parameters." The complete list of the eight nomograms and scenarios that appeared in the Insights Newsletter cited above and can be accessed at www.prostate-cancer.org.

Localized and Distant Metastases

In **Stage D** or the **N+ to M+** stages, the disease will be encountered in 20 percent of patients according to urologist Mark Austenfeld and colleagues. At this stage, the cancer has progressed to the regional lymph **nodes,** or onto the **N stage.** A CT scan and MRI would be able to detect larger tumours in the lymph nodes. A late stage D (or **M+ stages**) of cancer is the most serious type of malignancy since it has spread well beyond the lymph nodes and has **metastasized** to other parts of the body including the bones. Usually this staging of cancer is incurable and the patient may at some time experience the symptoms of pain in his hips, shoulders and lower back. Muscular weakness, loss of appetite and weight are other symptoms, often before any diagnosis is made. Some patients may not be feeling unwell even when diagnosed at a late stage of cancer progression. The radiation oncologist recommends the appropriate treatment but the chance of long-term survival for this patient is low. However, scientists are working diligently with new drugs and modern therapies for treating distant metastases. There is still much hope with the ever increasing research for extending a man's life, improving his quality of life, or for treating his pain, even when cancer has progressed beyond the pelvis region.

The five-year survival rate for patients with cancer in both N+ and M+ stages is estimated to be between 35 to 55 percent according to a study conducted by Dr. Zinner. Generally, hormonal therapy or orchiectomy (castration) would render potential benefits to patients with advanced prostate cancer. Patients at M1a to M1c staging are administered palliative therapy for suppressing the cancer or pain and any other discomforts when the need arises as the cancer progresses. Oncologists with specialized training are consulted for this kind of care. A man diagnosed with distant metastasis, or who is in a relapse after earlier treatment, would benefit from appropriate androgen deprivation therapy and chemotherapy. The relief from pain associated with bone cancer could be treated with new drugs such as biphosphonates and radiotherapy when cancer has metastasized in the bone as well as to further protect bones from the effects of the disease. Some clinics use radioactive 89strontium therapy given intravenously and this method of treatment may be able to prevent or curtail the growth of bone metastases. More research on treatment options will become available in the months and years ahead for treating advanced disease. Chapter 9 presents additional information on radiation therapy including hormonal and chemotherapy for advanced cancer patients.

What is a Cancer Grade?

There are three descriptive grades used to determine the shape, size and arrangement of cancerous or malignant cells which provide clues to the aggressive behaviour of prostate cancer. The three grades of cancer are defined as *well differentiated* (low grade), *moderately differentiated* (intermediate grade) and *poorly differentiated* (high grade). The Gleason scoring system ranges from 2-10 for the grading of prostate cancer tissues that establishes the activity of cancer growth. Dr. Donald Gleason identified *five different numerical patterns* of tumour tissues in his scheme. The Gleason grading scale (Figure 6.2) is ranked from 1 to 5, where 5 refers to poor cellular differentiation and is of the highest grade. The final Gleason score is found *by adding the grades of the two most common histological patterns from prostate tissues.* Well differentiated cells have a Gleason score of 2-4 by adding two grading patterns. A Gleason score of 5-6 represents moderately differentiated cancer cells (mild to moderately aggressive); a score of 7 shows moderately to poorly differentiated cancer cells, and a Gleason score of 8-10 represents definitive poorly differentiated cancer cells. Cancer cells that behave aggressively are likely to spread beyond the prostate capsule. Poorly differentiated cells appear and look very different to the clinician or pathologist from the well differentiated ones. Poorly differentiated cells are recognized as being fused into irregular and disorganized larger masses. Refer to the accompanying diagram of Gleason cancer patterns.

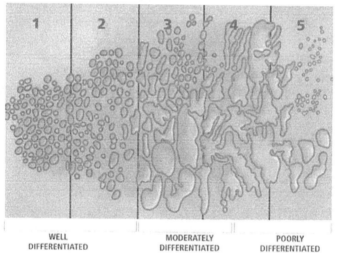

| WELL | MODERATELY | POORLY |
| DIFFERENTIATED | DIFFERENTIATED | DIFFERENTIATED |

Figure 6.2. The Gleason Grading System. Adapted with permission from AstraZeneca Canada.

The Gleason score or the sum is comprised of two grading patterns such as 2+3. The lowest Gleason score is found by adding the two lowest grades or 1+ 1 = 2, and the highest is 5+5 =10, thus the Gleason score ranges from 2 – 10. Gleason found that if he added the number of the *most common or predominant histological pattern* plus the s*econd most common pattern,* he would come up with a score such as 2 + 3 = 5 or 3 + 4 = 7. Gleason's reasoning was that a person who gets a biopsy has more than one malignant pattern. Take for example these two grades: 4 + 3 = 7 and 3 + 4 = 7. Both Gleason scores are 7 on the scale but the first grade of 4 of the former scenario, the most common pattern, behaves more aggressively than the grade of 3, a lower common grade. The second grade must be at least 5 percent the tumour volume that is evaluated by a pathologist. A study in Spain by Dr. Arbelaez Arango and colleagues analyzed cancer patients with Gleason scores of 3+4 and 4+3, and found that Gleason 4+3 patients had a higher serum PSA at diagnosis, greater surgical specimens, higher tumour volume, and had a tendency to present more advanced pathological stage than a Gleason of 3+4 cancers. When a Gleason score is determined it is important to know which number or grade is predominant or the preponderant histological pattern as seen under the microscope.

A Gleason score of 2 - 4 should indicate no seminal vesicle or lymph node invasion. Gleason scores of 8 - 10 are more likely to be associated with capsule penetration, lymph node invasion or seminal vesicle involvement. Most men diagnosed with prostate cancer fall in the middle of the Gleason system having scores of 5, 6, or 7. Dr. Pound and colleagues from Johns Hopkins reported on ten-year survivals after surgery without evidence of disease for increasing Gleason scores. A Gleason of 2 – 5, survival was 93 percent, and decreased to 78 percent for a Gleason of 6; survival was 46 percent for a Gleason of 7, and 23 percent for a Gleason of 8 – 10. The Partin and Sloan-Kettering nomograms would be a useful reference for patients when the Gleason scores and grades, PSA and staging are known – refer to the nomogram websites provided earlier in this chapter. Dr. Scardino cautions that Gleason patterns 1 and 2 may not be cancer at all; if a biopsy report indicates a Gleason score (not grade) of 5 or less, it warrants a review of the pathologist's report or microscopic slides; in other words, a second opinion is needed or the biopsy should be repeated in about three months. Treatment may not be necessary in the latter case. It is important for the patient to know the two grades of his cancer and the percent of his tumour. The one Gleason score, without knowing the two patterns provided in a biopsy report is not sufficient. In addition, it is important to realize that Gleason scores of 3+4 = 7 are very different than one of 5+2 = 7 or 4+3 = 7.

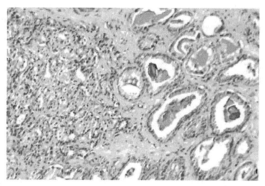

Figure 6.3: A microscopic slide (300x) showing pathology of Gleason grades. On the left is less normal tissue with a Gleason grade of 4 (out of 5) and highly undifferentiated. On the right is a Gleason grade of 3 with moderately differentiated cancer. Adapted from the National Cancer Institute Visuals.

The cancer grade, total and free PSA, cancer volume and stage of prostate cancer should all be known by the oncologist or urologist so as to determine the kind of treatment that is optimum for the patient. The number of positive biopsies provides important clues regarding the size of the tumour(s) and its volume. It is also important to have at least 6 to 8 biopsy core samples taken. If an individual is told that he has prostate cancer, he needs to be informed about all of his tests and to have them interpreted by his physician. My own cancer was at stage T2 and generally well differentiated before my surgery. After the surgery from the pathology report, one region of my prostate gland was found to be moderately differentiated following surgery. Most of my own prostate tissue was well differentiated. I felt that I was at a safe level and my cancer was not behaving aggressively. There is a correlation between the Gleason score and grade, and the number of needle biopsies *before* surgery, with the Gleason score and grade *after* radical prostatectomy. A 12-year study in Austria by Dr. Bektic and colleagues with 843 men separated into three groups by having 6, 10, and 15 core biopsies, were evaluated for congruency between initial needle biopsy and prostatectomy Gleason score. They found that taking 15 biopsy cores improved the concordance between initial biopsy and prostatectomy Gleason score to approximately 50 percent, reducing initial grading errors. The higher the number of the biopsy core samples taken before any treatment "the more accurate the treatment for patients with newly diagnosed prostate cancer." Dr. Freedland and colleagues noted that men with higher preoperative PSA concentrations had higher grade cancers and experienced the risk of bio-chemical progression. Although the total PSA value is very meaningful in detecting conditions of the prostate as well as tumour marker, the Gleason grade and the number of biopsy cores are more significant in diagnosing the extent of man's cancer or tumour(s). The *free PSA* percent in addition to the total PSA and DRE should be used in detecting prostate cancer and to make a decision on whether a biopsy is necessary.

Your doctor may appear not to have the time to provide all of the answers to your questions and some physicians may not have all of the answers at hand. One way to further investigate your specific concerns about prostate cancer and treatment options is to explore the appropriate internet sites listed in this book, acquire scientific and medical materials, and talk to other men in a prostate support group. Of course by reading this book, you are presented with second opinions, personal experiences and with updated information from the literature. If you are diagnosed with prostate cancer you will naturally be concerned as to whether your cancer is confined to the prostate or whether it has escaped the capsule. The oncologist and an urologist will interpret the data from your labora-tory tests and then establish a profile for you based on **your present health or any comorbidities, your age, DRE findings, your free and total PSA, PSA velocity or doubling time, your Gleason score and grades, how many positive biopsies were collected, tumour volume, a consideration of family history and your ethnic group**. You should be able to predict the extent of your prostate cancer to a high degree of accu-racy when your specialist explains the Partin Tables or Sloan-Kettering nomogram. Mathematical models use the data from tests to predict or gauge the extent of cancer and what may likely happen later. Take some time to access the websites provided and even plug in any hypothetical data to evaluate how those nomograms work. But as a patient, be fore-warned that the tables for the prediction of treatment options may not be representative of your own situation and it is important to consult with an urologist or oncologist. Treatment options provided in this chapter and others reflect the opinions of researchers in the literature and my person-al experiences as a patient who was diagnosed and treated for prostate cancer. This information is not meant to replace the advice of physicians and health care professionals.

Chapter 7

Radical Prostatectomy, Alternative Treatment Options, Concerns and Personal Experiences

By reading this chapter you will learn:

- About a decision to have a radical prostatectomy.
- How to prepare for surgery.
- Questions to ask your general practitioner, urologist or oncologist.
- Including your spouse or partner from diagnosis to post-treatment.
- Knowledge of your medical profile for optimum treatment, and review of nomograms.
- How is radical prostatectomy performed; my personal experiences.
- What you need to know following surgery.
- What are the risks and problems associated with surgery.
- Treating prostate cancer by laparoscopic prostatectomy, cryosurgery and high intensity focused ultrasound.

Getting Prepared

It is necessary to establish a profile of your present prostate and health condition based on the tests that have been taken. Your prostate profile may include the Gleason grade and score, the total and free PSA values, PSA velocity, TNM staging and DRE findings. The Partin algorithms are useful in predicting disease progression or risk assessment. Your age and health condition or any comorbidities upon diagnosis are important factors which should be considered in any treatment plan. If you smoke, stop, and if you are overweight it is recommended that you gradually lose any extra kilos to make the surgery easier for the surgeon and yourself. It is very important to gather as much information as possible on a variety of treatment options available from your urologist or oncologist when prostate cancer is first diagnosed. The first priority is for an optimum treatment and a cure. One suggestion is to further educate yourself about your health condition including the results of the tests once you have been diagnosed with prostate cancer. There is no immediate need to rush and have treatment since you have been living with your cancer for some time. It would be helpful to contact a community or provincial Prostate Support Group where you and your spouse or partner will meet with men who are either awaiting treatment or have been treated for prostate cancer, and who may have also experienced conditions like yours. Some support groups have contact with a staff of professionals at the Canadian Cancer Society or Cancer Agency who could also be of help in alleviating some of your concerns and fears. Some men at the support groups are quite knowledgeable about prostate cancer, having prior experiences with their diagnosis and treatment. Men in any support group are familiar with prostate cancer and their own medical situation but be cautious about any medical advice being suggested; medical advice should be provided by your doctor.

Things may not appear to be as bad when first hearing of the news of being diagnosed with prostate cancer. Of course, being told you have cancer is a shock. Some men and their spouses or partners may wish to receive counselling and other professional assistance that Cancer Clinics in each province provide. Do not hesitate to telephone the Cancer Clinic or the Canadian Cancer Society (CCS) and someone there will be able to provide assistance or direct you to the appropriate department or professional person. You may also contact the CCS or the Canadian Prostate Network at www.cpcn.org to locate support groups in your area. As mentioned above, men at the support groups are quite knowledgeable about their own condition and treatment, and are generally willing to share some of their own personal experiences. You should not isolate yourself after hearing the cancer diagnoses. Be willing to discuss any concerns with others, especially those who are close to you. Refer to Chapter 10 for ways to cope and deal with prostate cancer diagnosis.

You may wish to seek the opinion of another physician while anticipating treatment for prostate cancer. Good urologists and oncologists are difficult to find on your own and a patient generally takes the advice from his general practitioner for which specialist to consult through a referral system. The suggestion of getting another professional opinion poses some difficulty in Canada since it is almost impossible to find another urologist who is willing to accommodate the patient unless he wishes to wait for several more weeks for that appointment. Radiation oncologists generally work at a Cancer Clinic or hospital facility and do not have a private practice in Canada. It is normal to feel that way during the waiting period and anxious to get on with treatment. If you decide on getting a second opinion be sure not to consult with another urologist in the same medical group. After having some of your initial questions and concerns answered (and this process could take many weeks), it is ultimately your decision to consider on a particular treatment when you are satisfied that all or most of your questions have been answered. The decision for treatment should be guided by expert advice after consultation. Some people believe that doctors often provide the best advice and that the patient should generally follow his physician's treatment plan. General practitioners are generalists and may not always provide the same level of advice that is available from urologists and oncologists. If you decide on having radical prostatectomy, it is advisable to see an oncologist if only for another opinion and to answer your questions. Be cautious when seeking advice from non-professional individuals or from unreliable Internet sources. Expert medical advice is the primary goal for any cancer treatment. One website that is useful as a reference to combat any health-related frauds or fads is www.quackwatch.org. Refer to Chapter 11 for more information about this website.

Knowledge ultimately gives salvation, so you should try to be as well informed as possible before you make any decisions on a specific treatment option. You should also keep a personal medical file including a record of all of your visits to your physicians and the results of your tests. What did you last see your doctor for and what is the follow up plan? Think of as many questions that are relevant to your situation, diagnosis or impending treatment. I have provided a list of questions below for you to consider when you meet with your specialists or general practitioner. There is no such thing as a dumb question when it concerns your own health so do not be apprehensive to ask questions; your doctors are there to help you. Be honest with your doctor but you may have to ask questions about a course of a treatment, of any concerns and why a particular treatment is necessary. You are merely seeking clarification and more information. If you do not feel right about something, make it clear to your physician. Be open and frank. Be sure to take your written questions with you when you visit your urologist, oncologist or family physician. Make one copy for yourself and another for your physician. I did precisely that when I visited my urologist before my surgery. All my questions were answered and I felt mentally prepared for my surgery. Ask your spouse or a member of your family to accompany you, to gather and share information. It may be helpful to tape the discussion, with the doctor's permission. A physician you can trust makes this process easier.

Questions to Ask Your Doctors

The following are some useful questions that you may select and ask your **primary care physician, urologist or oncologist.** You may select which questions to ask on your first visit, then others on subsequent visits.

• Where precisely is my tumour located?

• To what stage do you think that my tumour has advanced?

• What is the grade of my cancer and the Gleason score? Please explain what it means.

• Did the pathologist provide the two Gleason grades (3+4 or 4+3)?

• Do you think that my cancer has left the prostate capsule or is it confined to the prostate gland? How can you tell?

• What is the extent of spreading or metastasis of my cancer?

• How many positive biopsies were found?

• For my age what should the PSA reading be if I had no cancer?

• What is my PSA reading now? What does this value indicate?

• Within one year do you have any idea how my cancer would progress if I opt to have no treatment now?

• What is the optimum treatment for me?

• I heard that the Partin tables and other nomograms could predict or assess my risk. Can you help me in this regard?

Questions To Ask Your Urologist

• How many of these operations have you performed in the past year?

• Can you give me the names and telephone numbers of three or four patients you have treated or can you arrange to have them call me?

• If surgery is the option, how would you do the operation - your procedure?

• What are the chances of being sexually potent after surgery? How do you carry out your nerve-sparing technique? Am I eligible for it?

• If my nerves cannot be spared can I have a nerve graft?

• How do you perform the surgery to prevent urinary stricture or incontinence?

• What is your success rate for incontinence and erectile dysfunction?

• Would I need a blood transfusion? What percent of your patients are not transfused? Can I donate my own blood ahead of time and how do I arrange for this?

• How do I prepare myself for the day of surgery or week before surgery?

• When is my surgery planned for? How long does the surgery last? How long would I have to stay in the hospital?

• Tell me about the catheter; how does it work? How do I look after it to prevent infections when I am discharged? How long do I have to keep it in after surgery?

• Do I need a bone scan or CT scan?

• What are the general procedures to follow before I am admitted for surgery?

• To ask following surgery: What was the grade of my cancer; was my cancer confined not; were the lymph nodes and seminal vesicles cancer free from the pathology report? (Get copies of your reports)

• How long will it be before I am fully cured of prostate cancer? What follow-up tests do I have to take?

• What are the chances of my cancer of this type recurring?

• If during the surgery my lymph nodes are positive for malignancy, what will be your plan of action?

• How are the Kegel exercises done? Can I have some information?

• How long will it take before I am sexually active again? Should I take any medication after surgery? When should I start on any modern drugs and what would you recommend?

• If hormonal manipulation is recommended what are the side effects of the drugs? What hormonal therapy are you recommending for me now?

• Can I have surgery without hormonal therapy? Why do I need to take hormones?

• What are the side effects of my medication or how would I react to the drug(s) you prescribed?

• If I have positive margins can I get an opinion about post-operative radiation therapy?

Questions to Ask Your Oncologist

• When do I start my treatment? Do I need hormonal therapy before radiation?

• How many treatments do I have to have? When will it be over?

• How long does each treatment last? What are the procedures?

• Can I drive home after each radiation treatment?

• Can I schedule my treatment around my work?

• What are the immediate side effects from radiation? What type of radiation therapy am I being put on? What kinds of foods or drinks should I avoid?

• What are the chances that my cancer will be eradicated?

• When do I have a repeat PSA? What should the PSA indicate after radiation?

• What are the long-term effects from the radiation?

• Can I have some literature on three-dimensional conformal radiation and intensity modulated radiation therapy? Which therapy will I have?

• What dose of radiation will I be getting?

• What is the "seed" implantation or brachytherapy procedure and how much more effective or less effective is it than external beam radiation? Is seed implantation an option for me? Why, why not?

• When would I see you again and can I see you during the course of my treatment if I am having problems?

• Do I have to take hormonal therapy after radiation? If so, for how long?

• If my cancer returns, what will be the next treatment option?

These sample questions can help you prepare for your treatment and in making the right decisions for controlling and/or providing a cure for your cancer. You will have your own specific questions to ask in addition to the ones provided above. The National Comprehensive Cancer Network in conjunction with the American Cancer Society provides second opinions on treatment options by logging on to www.nccn.org. The Partin and Narayan Tables through a Google search or at www.prostate-cancer.org/ provide a second opinion on treatment options when the patient has information to provide. As mentioned in Chapter 6, the nomogram developed by Memorial Sloan-Kettering (www.mskcc.org/mskcc/html/10088.cfm) is also useful in planning ahead or for predicting the progression of disease. You should insist on having an explanation for your concerns before you walk out of the physician's office and know what you are expected to do before your next visit. It may be some time before you will see your physician again. Make written notes of your concerns during the meeting with your doctor, including your physician's responses. Your spouse or a family member may also act as your secretary during this visit, taking notes and asking questions you may have missed. Another suggestion is to rehearse the interview process with your partner, spouse or a friend before your appointment.

After the Biopsy

A bone scan may be recommended by the urologist or oncologist if malignancy is detected. A ProstaScint scan may be done to determine if cancer has moved to the lymph nodes (see Chapter 9). This test may not very effective in identifying all nodal cancers. Stages A and B cancers (T1b to T2c) will not likely show any metastases in the bones but your physician can order one for you as added assurance that all is well. Urologist Scardino noted that it is uncommon for cancer to register on a bone scan if the PSA is less than 20 and extremely rare with a PSA under 8. In one study of 306 men with a PSA score of less than 20, only one patient had a positive metastasis of a bone scan. Ask about the procedure, if one is recommended. The bone scan procedure uses a special type of X-ray made by first injecting the patient with a radioactive substance that highlights areas of the skeletal tissues or bones. When I had my bone scan done I was first injected with a radioactive substance and had to return some two hours later for the actual bone scan procedure. It takes some time for the radionuclide substance to circulate through the bloodstream. A gamma ray camera records where the radionuclide accumulates. The procedure takes about twenty minutes and the patient experiences no dis-comfort. I was anxious to see my results when the nuclear medical spe-cialist came in to check on the computer monitor where I saw my skele-ton in living colour. I asked him for details of the scan, if there were any progression of my cancer but he gave me a reassuring smile which I took as negative for cancer; he could not give me the results as that would not be following protocol.

When someone is in a life-threatening situation and anxious to know the results of tests and is denied the opportunity, it makes little sense not to inform patients as soon as possible. Would it not have been better to take that opportunity to explain the bone scan which I saw in front of me? Instead, I had to wait for another week to see my urologist for the results. I was learning to become very patient. Yes, frustration does accumulate so patients should be reminded of some of the "inconveniences" during the waiting period. My cancer fortunately had not metastasized into my bone. Bone cancer shows up as "hot spots" mainly along the ribs, spine, skull and pelvis regions.

Another procedure which may be considered is the computerized tomography scan or CT scan and provides cross-sectional images of the body. This procedure is done for a high Gleason grade and score, an elevated PSA with the patient having several positive biopsies that are suspicious for extra-capsular prostate cancer or for any advanced TNM staging. The patient is injected with an intravenous dye and the results from the test become available in a couple of days; be aware that some men may be allergic to the dye. The CT scan may be able to determine if any cancer has moved to the lymph nodes. The MRI or magnetic resonance imaging is not done for detecting prostate cancer but for pelvic lymph node evaluation and for men who are at very high risk. These procedures are not recommended for diagnosing prostate cancer. However the ProstaScint and MRI imaging "significantly enhance detection of nodal disease....and provide information to help design treatment fields and to optimize existing fields for radiotherapy" according to research by Dr. Kipper. The ProstaScint scan involves a radioactive isotope attached to an antibody that seeks out that specific prostate cancer protein. The patient returns four days later to be scanned by a gamma ray camera. The procedure may be able to diagnose seminal vesicle and lymph node cancer and to determine ahead of time what treatment is needed. ProstaScint scanning is not routinely used and may not be totally reliable.

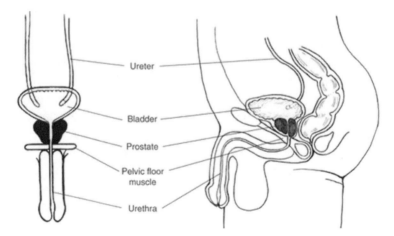

Figure 7.1: Front and side views of the Male Genitourinary System. Adapted from the National Institute of Diabetes and Digestive and Kidney Diseases, the National Institute of Health.

Radical Prostatectomy and a Retrospective View

There is a high probability of cure after a radical prostatectomy if the following four criteria are met: (a) the cancer is localized and confined to the prostate gland at stages T1 to T2c; (b) the cancer grade is well to moderately differentiated; (c) the PSA is less than 4.0, and (c) the person is in general good health. With stages T1a through to T2, in order to achieve 100 percent curative treatment, the tumour must be confined to the prostate and has not escaped the margin of the prostate. By opting for surgery, the entire prostate is removed and, if possible, every effort is made to spare the two neurovascular bundles responsible for erectile potency and to leave the external sphincter muscle (see pelvic floor muscle in Figure 7.1) intact to reduce the incidence of incontinence. Nerve-sparing technique may not be possible with every surgical procedure. The hands and experience of the surgeon are of utmost importance as the surgery is very delicate with the primary goal being to remove all the cancer. Nerve grafts for restoring sexual potency may not be necessary if the surgeon is experienced and the cancer is confined to the prostate gland. Even when a nerve graft is done, it may not necessarily restore erectile potency. Dr. Walsh, the pioneer of the nerve-sparing radical prostatectomy, pointed out that "the neurovascular bundles are located at an average of 4.9 mm away from the prostate" and even with some capsular penetration of cancer the nerves can still be spared. The secondary goals of surgery are to prevent any long-term incontinence by saving the external sphincter muscle, as well as the two neurovascular bundles. Dr. Freedland and investigators in a study of over 7 000 men who were treated by seven experienced surgeons found that obesity or body mass index was positively related to capsular incision. An intact prostate gland following radical prostatectomy is desirable and keeps any cancer cells from escaping.

You should ask to have a copy of the reports from your urologist and pathologist following surgery when you visit your family physician or urologist and to review how your surgery was performed and whether there were any complications. You should ask for an interpretation of the written reports and keep copies for future reference. You have a right to know all your test results and to receive an explanation from your doctor. I asked my physician for copies of the reports from my urologist and pathologist. I have always kept a record of my tests and medical reports even before my diagnosis of prostate cancer. I certainly wanted to know about those lymph nodes and the extent of my cancer within the prostate as well as my final Gleason score and grade. Many patients, including some friends of mine, never ask for an explanation of their tests or medical reports from their doctor. Some doctors never explain what some of the test results mean to their patients. You must insist on seeing the results of any tests and ask for an explanation or interpretation. For example: What does a PSA of 2.4 mean for my age and should I be concerned about that level now? When should I have another PSA done? Why is this necessary? What was my PSA last year and what is its velocity since the last test? Do I need to have a biopsy done and if so when? Can I request a free PSA test including a total PSA test? What does a Gleason score of 6 tell me? These are only a few of the many questions you may ask depending on what tests or treatment options are suggested or taken. Don't take "it's good" or "nothing to worry about" as answers from your doctor when enquiring about your test results.

Before and After the Scalpel

The day before my surgery I had to follow a liquid only diet and all solids had to be removed from my bowels. Surgery was scheduled for eight the next morning. The night before an anesthetist visited me when I was at the hospital and asked me a number of questions. He was very thorough and I felt that he ought to be the one to put me out! The next morning, after a good night's sleep, I was ready for the big day. I was actually excited to get on with the surgery, wanting to rid my body of the cancer. Promptly at eight in the morning, a male nurse took me down the elevator to the OT; that's the abbreviation for the operating theatre, I later learned. Somewhere between OT and my room I was shaved by that efficient male nurse and I recalled asking him if he ever made a mistake with using his sharp razor. He did not seem to be too amused by my sense of humour even at that crucial hour.

Moments later I was in the OT and was happy to see my primary care physician wearing a surgical mask and ready to assist my urologist. My memory flashed back to about six months earlier when my doctor found that lump through DRE. He had told me that he would be there to assist the surgeon. It was very comforting for me to have him assist my urologist during the surgery because he discovered my tumour and I continue to have complete trust and faith in him as my primary care physician. It was also comforting to know that I was in good hands with my urologist. I was ready for the scalpel. I had researched my urologist and discovered he was a very good surgeon, trained at Memorial Sloan-Kettering. That was good, because very soon he was going to remove my organ-confined cancerous prostate gland. My surgery was a retropubic radical prostatectomy procedure. Sometimes perineal radical prostatectomy may be carried out, especially in cases of abdominal obesity.

At first I did not recognize my primary care doctor wearing his surgical mask until he asked me for a telephone number of a close relative that my urologist would contact after my surgery. I gave him my son's work number. I then wondered why they needed an emergency number. Thoughts of not making it through the surgery ran briefly through my mind. Confidence in my urologist was again my primary focus even though he had not dissected rats in high school biology. As I glanced over to one side of the OT I saw my urologist chatting nonchalantly with another colleague; two female nurses wearing surgical masks while waiting expressionless for me to "go under" stood around the huge lamps in the OT. I wanted some sort of reassuring smile to keep my spirits up for that brief moment. The anesthetist who came to see me the night before told me what he was going to do with my IV. I recognized him again, then he asked me to count to ten. I faintly remember making the count to seven!

I later read the Operative Procedure Report about my retropubic radical prostatectomy. I could picture myself being draped in the supine position and my urologist's steady and experienced hand making the first incision just from the left side of my belly button. Having been shaven and disinfected in the area, a midline incision was made, skirting the umbilicus (the navel region) just to the left side and it continued straight down above the pubic bone region in the pelvic region. I recall that the surgery was going to be a retropubic one and that it was not an easy surgery to perform by any inexperienced surgeon because the prostate gland is located deep within the pelvis and surrounded by blood vessels, nerves, sphincter muscles that must be saved for complete success. I should add that the healed incision, 15 cm in length, looked perfectly straight except for the small incision that skirted around my navel area. My abdominal muscles were separated during the procedure and were spread apart after the incision was made. Surgical retractors were used to keep the abdominal tissues apart so as to allow for a good view of the bladder, prostate and pelvic lymph nodes. Two lymph nodes were removed, one from each side of my pelvic area, and sent to the pathology lab for analysis before my surgeon would proceed with removing my entire prostate gland. Lymph nodes are quickly frozen for slicing before microscopic analysis. Fortunately, both nodes revealed no malignancy and the surgery was able to continue. Had those nodes been cancerous, my urologist would have terminated the surgery. Unfortunately, the patient does not have a say at that moment on whether to proceed or not with surgery if lymph nodes were positive for cancer. You may want to discuss that important option before having surgery – whether to continue or to abort the surgery. I wondered what my physicians and nurses were doing or saying while waiting for the pathologist's report on those lymph nodes!

The prostate gland was carefully isolated to view the urethra and neurovascular bundles. My urethra was mobilized during the delicate surgery leaving intact the two neurovascular bundles on the right and left sides of the prostate. The two neurovascular bundles carry both nerves and blood vessels alongside the prostate. The major dorsal vein system was divided and tied. I could visualize my urologist using his best skills with his scalpel and other instruments. My surgeon had removed my cancerous prostate gland, saved the external sphincter muscle for preventing incontinence and spared my nerves for restoring sexual potency.

Sexual potency may be restored through nerve-sparing surgery but not always. It may be possible to do a nerve graft that could improve the chances of restoring sexual potency if the nerves had to be severed; the procedure may require the hands of a nerve graft expert but some urologists are also trained in this procedure. An incision was made at the base of the prostate close enough to save the sphincter muscles around the urethra. My prostate gland was removed by a sharp incision at the base of the bladder neck. The surgical procedure was a very delicate one as an incision too close to the prostate gland may leave some cancer behind. My urethra was therefore shortened as a small piece of it was removed together with my prostate gland. The urologist may test the carvernous nerves with a neurostimulator for its potential function. The lower side of my intact urethra was later sutured to the base of the bladder, a process physicians refer to as an anastomosis. The surgeon rebuilds the urethra by suturing the sphincter end of the urethra that was below the prostate gland onto the base of the bladder. The bladder, being mobile, is pulled down to join with the urethra during the anastomosis procedure. The urologist then checks that the connection between the bladder neck and urethra is water-tight. The dorsal vein complex that was earlier cut and tied was then sutured together. During the surgery my two seminal vesicles were also removed; this seems to be the normal routine procedure during a radical prostatectomy. To ensure that no cancerous cells remain, those two semi-nal vesicles were rendered useless and were excised even without any capsular penetration. There will be no more seminal fluids and I will remain sterile. However, with a dry ejaculate, sexual potency was restored.

I "tolerated the procedure well" was one written comment in my urol-ogist's report. There were no complications during the surgery with a loss 600 ml. of blood; I was fortunately not transfused. I still continue to have a 99 percent faith on the quality of blood supply by the Red Cross. After the anastomosis was completed an "18 French 30 cc Foley catheter" (Figure 7.3) was placed into my penis, then inserted into the urethra through to the bladder neck opening and anchored by a tiny balloon into the bladder. The catheter was hooked up to a bag externally which I was to wear for the next three weeks; some urologists recommend one to two weeks duration for wearing the catheter. The skin clips or staples that held the incision together after the surgery were removed five days after sur-gery and before I was discharged. Two drains (small tubes) were placed on the right and left side of my incision into my abdominal region to remove any excess fluids that build up; removing them before I was dis-charged was a more unpleasant experience than getting the staples out from my incision. The accompanying diagrams illustrate how retropubic and perineal radical prostatectomy are accomplished.

What about that malignant prostate gland? I understand that India ink is used to coat the gland and then a fixative is added before it is sectioned and stained for microscopic examination. The findings from the patholo-gy report about my surgery read in part: "The prostate gland measured 4 x 2.5 cm in transverse diameters and is 2.0 cm in length. The specimen now weighs 14.0 grams" and it seemed that the hormone therapy I took weeks before had reduced the size of my prostate gland. I am not con-vinced, however, that my cancer was downgraded by hormone therapy. The report of my surgery and pathology continued as follows: "There is no grossly identifiable tumor. Sections of right and left pelvic lymph

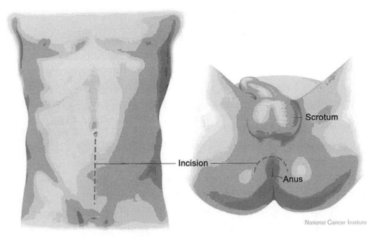

Figure 7.2: The dotted lines indicate where incisions are made for radical retropubic prostatectomy on the left, and on the right for perineal prostatectomy. Adapted from the National Cancer Institute Visuals.

nodes show no evidence of malignancy. Sections of the radical prostatectomy specimen show moderately differentiated prostate adenocarcinoma in sections taken from the right lateral and posterior lobes; this involves less than 10 percent of the prostatic tissue; the tumour was well differentiated." My Gleason grade was 3 in the moderately differentiated tissue specimen and my "malignancy extended to within 1.0 mm of the capsular margin and capsular transgression was not identified."

As for the seminal vesicles, they were also free of malignancy. From the pathologist's report I believe that I should be free of prostatic cancer. But for how many years? I kept wondering. It was indeed a real close call, with only one millimetre left before cancer cells would have penetrated the prostate capsule and gone into adjacent tissues. Am I out of the woods yet? My urologist prescribed periodic PSA tests told me to see him for the next few years. More than 12 years have passed since my surgery was performed. I have had more than 12 PSA tests to check for any recurrent disease. My PSA reading has been less than 0.04 ug/l using the Immulite 2000 assay and consistent from the same laboratory. Before my surgery my PSA was 0.2 ug/l – a false negative reading. I may have something to celebrate now since there seems to be no recurrent disease! Hopefully all of my cancer is gone. My general practitioner recently assured me that I should have nothing to worry about.

Laparoscopic Prostatectomy

A surgical technique that is being done in recent years and growing in popularity is *laparoscopic prostatectomy,* and carried out by a few experienced surgeons. Surgeons in Paris at one facility have been performing that procedure for prostate cancer for several years with much success. The procedure uses a lighted tube that enters the body through tiny openings that allow the surgeon to manipulate the microsurgical instrument. Earlier studies reported that the incidence of common problems such as erectile dysfunction in post-surgery seem to be similar for open prostatectomy procedure. Some surgeons also perform laparoscopic surgery by the use of a robotic interface which uses more delicate instruments than laparoscopic hand surgery. The surgeon maneuvers instruments via a computer interface for robotic laparoscopy. The experience of using robotic laparoscopy for radical prostatectomy is more common with European surgeons than with North American surgeons at this time. The surgical procedure lasts for about 1.5 to 2 hours and the patient experiences less pain, less loss of blood, comparable recovery from incontinence and sexual dysfunction as with open radical prostatectomy done by experienced surgeons. According to urologist Scardino at Memorial Sloan-Kettering, his colleague Dr. Guillonneau has been very successful in conducting hundreds of laparoscopic radical prostatectomy procedures; of his latest experience with 250 patients, the rate of positive margins was 10 percent and 53 percent of men regained erections at three months without any medication.

At Johns Hopkins University, Drs. Su and Pavlovich have been performing laparoscopic surgery using robotic technique for several years on hundreds of patients. Dr. Walsh questions whether laparoscopic prostatectomy will ever be as effective as the "gold standard" of open radical retropubic prostatectomy. He contends that with open surgery, the hands of the surgeon directly in contact with the structures in and around the prostate have an added advantage. Several clinics in Canada routinely perform laparoscopic surgery for removal of gall bladders and other minor surgeries. Laparoscopic prostatectomy is now being performed at McGill University in Montreal as well as in Hamilton, Toronto, Regina and Edmonton. At the London Health Sciences Centre in Ontario, a state-of-the-art technology, the robotic *da Vinci* surgical system developed by Canadian Surgical Technologies & Advanced Robotics (CSTAR) performs cardiac and urology surgery. Dr. Joseph Chinn is one of the urologists who operates the da Vinci robot's 3-dimensional imaging that provides better visual magnification resulting in greater surgical accuracy. CSTAR reduces the risk of stroke or clot formation on patients suffering from atrial fibrillation.

Following Surgery

Immediately following surgery and after regaining consciousness, my first recollection was of being in a room that was being kept very cold and that nurses were keeping me warm with blankets. The temperature in the operating room was lower than normal in order to reduce any bacterial or viral infections during surgery. Sometime following surgery I was taken back to my room on the fourth floor of the Royal Columbian Hospital in New Westminister, British Columbia, and where on a happier occasion in 1965 my daughter was born. I slept well following surgery because I had no recollections of the rest of the day and only vaguely late in the evening I started to become aware of my surroundings. The day following surgery I was encouraged to walk so as to increase my muscle movements in order to reduce any possible risk of blood clot formation. Taking a few steps was very difficult do as I had been experiencing a fair amount of abdominal pain from the surgery but I was able to self-administer my pain medication by intravenous means or IV; the latter is medically referred to as a patient-controlled analgesia and given through my intravenous fluid line. About five days following surgery I was discharged and I thank those hard-working and caring nurses on Ward Four North at the New Westminister Royal Columbian Hospital for their kindness and professional care.

Like most men, it felt quite uncomfortable wearing the catheter for that period of three weeks after surgery. I realized that it was part of my healing process and that I ought to be patient. Some men have reported bleeding around the catheter. See your doctor if any problems develop. Drinking lots of fluids that may help stop any minor bleeding; you should not needlessly worry about a tinge of blood. Some leakage around the catheter may also occur when having a bowel movement or even while walking around. But if the catheter is clogged or even dislodged call your doctor immediately and rush to the emergency of the closest hospital. After my catheter was removed I did not experience any lasting incontinence but after about two weeks while recuperating at home, I developed a urinary stricture or bladder neck contracture. I had another catheter inserted in place at the hospital's emergency when I had experienced closure of the bladder neck – during that time my urine flow was a mere trickle and I felt that my bladder was about to rupture while waiting for another catheter to be inserted to relieve the pressure. I was fortunate that I took quick action and was driven to the same hospital where my surgery was done, not far from my home. I was beginning to wonder how long I would have to wear the catheter and what was I getting into with this new development of urinary stricture! I felt that things were moving along quite smoothly with my post-operation until this urinary condition developed.

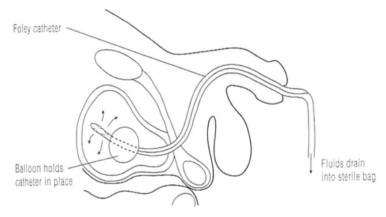

Figure 7.3: Foley Catheter inserted into the penis. This illustration was adapted from the Kidney & Urologic Diseases Information Clearinghouse, National Institute of Health.

Some days later my urologist used the cystoscope to investigate the cause of my urinary stricture. The cystoscope procedure went fairly well; I remember the procedure from before my surgery. A tube with a tiny light source is inserted into the penis that courses its way up the urethra. Another instrument resembling cystoscope, a metal catheter called a "sound" was used to cut through the base of my bladder and it created more discomfort and pain than the cystoscope procedure. I later wondered why my urologist did not use a local anesthetic for this minor surgery of removing a piece of scar tissue he said was blocking my bladder neck that caused my urinary stricture – that latter minor surgical procedure is referred to as internal urethrotomy. Bladder neck contracture or stricture has been reported on an average of 4.8 percent following surgery according to Dr. Strum. Experienced surgeons average about 1 percent strictures with their patients; strictures are rare after radical laparoscopic prostatectomy according to Dr. Scardino. Urinary stricture of my type was perhaps preferable, as I rationalized later, than having any prolonged incontinence! My urine flow had improved considerably since that minor but unpleasant surgery. Regarding incontinence, most patients seem to recover from it after several weeks or within a few months.

The complete recovery period after retropubic radical prostatectomy could take several weeks and most men are fully recovered after two months. Some physical discomfort may be experienced during the first few weeks following surgery and can include abdominal pain, diarrhea, constipation and fatigue. The physician and nursing staff are there to assist the patient to overcome any difficulties and provide the necessary medication the patient is discharged. When you are ready to resume work you should consult with your doctor. You should not be in any rush to return to work and should be well rested, especially if strenuous physical activity is part of your daily work. A home care nurse visited me while I was wearing the catheter. Infections can develop if you do not use a disinfectant or clean the rubber tubing around the penis area. I was eagerly awaiting the end of the three weeks of wearing that "appendage" but had to settle for an additional few more weeks after my trouble with the urinary stricture.

I was able to walk to the grocery and drive my car for short distances while wearing the catheter. I tried not to let it bother me as I realized that I had to live with it for a while and that it was in my best interest to tolerate it during my second healing period. As a matter of fact, I asked my urologist if I could go on a vacation while wearing my catheter after he had taken care of the urinary stricture, knowing that I would have to look after it and have the bag strapped to my thigh or leg while away. He said that it should not be a problem to travel. I felt that I was gaining my strength and I had a positive outlook on life, knowing that the report on my surgery was good. I later took a three-day vacation to my favorite city, San Francisco, and had an eventful time. I experienced no problems getting on and off those cable cars and walking around Fishermans's Wharf.

I even took the BART and visited several sites including Berkeley University.

During the first year following my surgery I saw my urologist a few times. About four months after surgery, I had my first PSA test done to see if any residual disease was present. Your PSA test should be done after three to four months following surgery or radiation. My PSA before the biopsy was 0.2 ug/l and it was a false negative before having my surgery because my tumour was well differentiated and very small. I therefore did not expect any rise in PSA following surgery but we will never know the outcome of surgery even after several years. My PSA today is less than 0.04 ug/l, more than 12 years after having radical prostatectomy. In theory, there should be no elevation of serum PSA if all the cancerous tissue was removed. Elevated PSA to detectable levels suggests recurrence of disease after surgery; if that is the case then local radiotherapy on the prostate bed may be recommended but only if the cancer is believed to be still in the pelvic region. Hormonal therapy may also be given before, during and after radiation therapy. Chapter 9 discusses both radiotherapy and hormonal therapy.

Ask your nurses any questions you want – about what you can do, what you should not do, anything that comes to your mind. You probably would have asked your urologist questions following surgery. Avoid becoming constipated by taking stool softeners. Consult physician about medications. Your rectum was under some stress after surgery and had become tender; do not take any enemas during that time. Avoid lifting anything heavier than a telephone directory, avoid strenuous exercise, tennis, golf, riding a bike or horse, or jogging and avoid any lengthy walking at a strenuous pace. A walk is a good idea, but sit and rest every few hundred metres and when you return home. Increase on your daily walk; if you feel up to it, you should be able to drive your car for short distances after about three weeks. In about two to three months you will be able to swing that golf club again.

Dr. Michael Stuart reported in the *JAMA* on the risks and problems associated with having radical prostatectomy. In a 1992 study, Dr. Stuart noted that there was a 1-2 percent mortality rate, 25 percent impotence or erectile dysfunctional rate, 18 percent urinary stricture, a 6 percent risk of incontinence and a 3 percent risk of rectal injury after surgery. Data will change depending on which study is cited. Mortality rates, rectal injuries, urinary stricture, and incontinence are reported at lower rates in better-care facilities and with surgeon experience. The rates of erectile dysfunction after surgery is often reported to be much higher than the 25 percent cited above even after one year following surgery. The next chapter discussed erectile dysfunction and treatment options in detail. The noted urologist William Catalona, in one study, reported that following radical prostatectomy the incidence of erectile dysfunction ranged from 30 to 60 percent; the incidence of incontinence was from 5 percent to 15 percent, rectal injury rate was from 0.1 to 7 percent, the death rate was from 0.15 to 2 percent, and the average blood loss was 0.5 to 2 litres. Dr. Lu-Yao raised major concerns about the increasing rate of radical prostatectomy in men 75 years and older in the U.S. Of 10 598 radical prostatectomy operations studied by Dr. Lu-Yao, 2 percent of men aged 75 and older died and nearly 8 percent suffered major cardio-pulmonary complications with 30 days of the operation.

Your urologist should discuss with you any potential risks involved before you decide on surgery. There are conflicting views and arguments of whether a man older than 75 years of age should opt have surgery. There seems to be a dramatic increase rate of radical prostatectomy procedures on men between 60-79 years of age within the past 10 years in the North American population and especially in the United States. The full benefits derived from surgery in older men have not yet been determined; furthermore, surgery for men over 75 years of age has been questioned by many in the medical profession in Canada and elsewhere. Instead of choosing surgery, other alternative treatment options are available for an older man including hormone therapy, radiation therapy or objectified active surveillance. Factors such as a person's health, grade of cancer, the number of positive biopsies and PSA level would determine which treatment plan is best. Dr. Albertsen and colleagues estimated the survival rates of men 55 to 74 years of age with clinically localized prostate cancer diagnosed between 1971 and 1984; treatment was with androgen withdrawal therapy or by observation or no treatment. The study of 767 men was conducted before 1990 and reported in 1998 in *JAMA*. Men were separated into Gleason scores of 2-4, 5, 6, 7 and 8-10. Men with a Gleason score of 2-4 disease faced a minimal risk of death from prostate cancer within 15 years of diagnosis with conservative management. Men with a Gleason score of 8-10 had a 60 to 87 percent chance of dying from prostate cancer within 15 years. Those men with Gleason scores of 5-7 face a modest risk of death and increased over at least 15 years of follow-up. Survival rates declined with increasing Gleason scores and with conservative treatment. In 2005, Dr. Albertsen discussed the 20-year outcomes following conservative management of clinically localized prostate cancer from the above study. Men with low-grade prostate cancer have a small risk of cancer progression even after 20 years of management by androgen withdrawal or by observation and aggressive treatment was not recommended.

Cryosurgery

Cryotherapy is the freezing of the prostate gland to kill cancer cells using cryoprobes to deliver a temperature of -40°C; this procedure has improved over the years but there are some disadvantages as well as advantages with having cryotherapy. Over 500 patients were treated at the Crittenton Hospital in Rochester, Michigan, using cryotherapy procedures. There seems to be a reportedly high success rate with cryotherapy among patients having confined prostate cancer and relapse after radiation therapy. Of patients who had confined prostate cancer and after three years following cryosurgery, 10 percent had positive biopsies at the Rochester Hospital and this figure compares favourably with either post-radical prostatectomy or following external beam radiation. Dr. Bahn and his colleagues stated that the overall biopsy proven disease free rate was 85.8 percent in their study of 590 consecutive patients. Cryoablation or cryotherapy is done by circulating freezing argon gas with multiple cryoprobes guided by transrectal ultrasound and using multiple hollow blunt metallic thermocouples through the perineum or the region between the scrotum and anus. The procedure is similar to brachytherapy and the patient is under spinal anesthetic. Thermocouples monitor the temperature of surrounding tissues and to ensue that adequate freezing is done on the prostate. The cryoprobes delivering argon are controlled by a computer. The prostate is frozen but the urethra and rectal area are protected from being frozen by circulating warm water with a lubricated catheter through the penis into the bladder. Before any freezing is done, sterile saline solution is injected between the rectal wall and the prostate gland for added protection. The specialist doing the procedure must be aware of an ice ball forming on the entire prostate gland so as to monitor how much freezing is required and when to stop the procedure. The procedure is repeated to ensure that the cancer is destroyed. The subsequent thawing of the frozen prostate helps kill cancer cells. After freezing is over and the surgeon is sure that the prostate gland has been frozen to kill the cancer cells, helium is circulated through the probes to thaw the prostate.

Proponents of cryotherapy like Drs. Katz and Bahn at Rochester said in a *Prostate Cancer Research Institute* report that cryoablation is "comparable to the rates of efficacy of both beam radiation and brachytherapy…and appears to be superior in the treatment of high risk disease." Dr. Bahn noted that cryotherapy today shows "promising modality in patients who are radiation therapy failures." Cryotherapy may also be used as a salvage procedure after brachytherapy for recurrent cancer. Dr. Bahn and colleagues are convinced that physicians and patients will find greater acceptance and utilization of cryotherapy as a primary treatment option for localized prostate cancer. One major disadvantage of cryotherapy is the high rate of erectile dysfunction from nerve damage; in one study 15 percent regained potency and additional 23 percent of men claimed partial recovery. The rate of urinary incontinence was low and less than 5 percent. It may take a few more years to know the true efficacy of cryotherapy for treating localized prostate cancer as well as to make better informed treatment comparisons between radiation and radical prostatectomy. In Canada, at the time of writing, cryotherapy procedures are being conducted in Calgary and in London, Ontario.

High Intensity Focused Ultrasound (HIFU)

High Intensity Focused Ultrasound (HIFU) is a new method under investigation in North America to destroy cancerous prostate tissue and to treat BPH using extreme heat generated by high-energy ultrasound waves. The high ultrasound creates a temperature of 80–90° Celsius. HIFU was first used to treat BPH and is at a pioneering stage in treating prostate cancer in North America but not in Europe. At the Don Mills Surgical Unit in Toronto, urologist John Warner who is the Medical Director of HIFU, works in conjunction with other outstanding urologists in Canada, are offering the *Ablatherm Maple Leaf HIFU* in their pioneering work in Canada. Information of HIFU in Canada is at www.hifu.ca. Studies in Europe suggest that HIFU may have a role in treating small and confined prostate cancers. It has been successfully used to treat over 7 000 patients in Europe. HIFU is also approved in England, France, Germany and

Japan. The patient is given a spinal anesthesia and an ultrasound probe is placed into the rectum so that the entire gland can be properly imaged. The surgeon selects the specific zone(s) for treatment by using computer imaging. The surgeon then begins the treatment and stops when the entire gland has been treated; the intensity and duration of therapy is determined by computer or can be operated manually. A single procedure lasts from 1.5 to 3.0 hours. The patient is fitted with a catheter after HIFU as bladder discomfort is common and the urethra experiences a certain amount of stress. Urologist Chinn wrote in the *Insights Newsletter* in 2004 and cautioned that there are some limitations to HIFU use; prostates larger than 40 cc may be downsized by hormonal therapy before treatment. The focal length of HIFU is also limited for prostate sizing. Potency and continence rates appear higher than that of post-surgery but more data is needed to confirm these findings. It was reported that rectal injuries appear to be of little concern with HIFU treatment.

Dr. Gelet and colleagues from France, reporting in *The Journal of Urology*, provided preliminary results of HIFU on 50 patients with localized prostate cancer who were not suitable candidates for radical prostatectomy. The results suggest that HIFU is a valid alternative treatment strategy for patients with localized prostate cancer patients who are unsuitable for surgery. Dr. Gelet claims that the use of HIFU as salvage therapy for locally recurrent prostate cancer after radiation therapy is advantageous. HIFU can be also be used as salvage therapy for radical prostatectomy according to Dr. Chinn. Both Drs. Poissonnier and Gelet found that in a study of 106 patients with local recurrence of prostate cancer after external beam radiation, and with salvage HIFU, the treatment provided a curative chance for patients with local recurrence, leading to favourable risk-benefit ratio compared with other types of salvage therapies. On the other hand, oncologist Pickles and colleagues in an article in the *Canadian Journal of Urology* noted that with HIFU the "lack of efficacy data does not allow meaningful assessment as to the benefit – risk ratio of HIFU treatment. It would therefore be inappropriate to offer HIFU as standard therapy for prostate cancer." Rectal fistula appears to be the most serious potential complication and over 50 percent rate of impotence has been reported with HIFU. Dr. Scardino cautions that since most cancers are multifocal or present in several places in the prostate, HIFU imaging techniques are unable to pinpoint all of the cancer clusters. Pickles and colleagues noted that not all of the tumours in the gland were destroyed by HIFU when patients were followed by radical prostatectomy and subsequent pathology. However, for older men who want to avoid surgery, cryotherapy or HIFU could be alternative treatment options. In my opinion, brachytherapy would be my first option for localized prostate cancer if I wanted to avoid surgery. Urologist Chinn explains that with the advanced HIFU technology, the incidence of rectal fistula was less than one percent and erectile dysfunction reported lower rates than previously stated. HIFU equipment such as the Ablatherm and Sonoblate 500 systems are expensive and require extensive training by the technician and surgeon. Consultation and research by prospective patients are highly recommended before undergoing HIFU treatment for confined prostate cancer.

The Europeans seem to have more data on HIFU since it has been in use from the early 1990s. Dr. Blana and colleagues in Germany reported on a five-year result of Ablatherm HIFU treatment on 146 patients. They found that 87 percent of patients had a constant PSA of less than 1.0 ng/ml and 93 percent of all patients had negative biopsies on follow up. The rate of erectile dysfunction was high but 47 percent of the patients had regained erectile potency according to their study. In March 2005, the National Institute for Health and Clinical Excellence (NICE) in Britain issued guidance to doctors using HIFU for prostate cancer. NICE concluded this treatment is safe enough providing men know what is involved and its side effects. The message to patients is to gather as much information about any treatment option and to be informed about proven treatment options before considering alternative options for treating prostate cancer with lack of efficacy data.

Summary

Your prostate profile should be known when considering any effective treatment options for prostate cancer. In general terms and in my opinion, if cancer is confined to the prostate and you are in good health, with a cancer grade that is well to moderately differentiated, with a PSA value of less than 5 at an age of 45-65 years, and in addition, with a PSA value of less than 10 at an age of 65 to about 70 years, then you might want to consider having radical prostatectomy or brachytherapy as your primary treatment options. If your life expectancy is less than 10 years or if you are 75 years or older with the conditions described above, having surgery may not be your best option even with low grade and confined prostate cancer. You may want to consider active surveillance. Your doctor will advise you on which option is best for your condition.

One Japanese study conducted by Dr. Tomita and colleagues in Tokyo of men aged 51 to 70 years of age and men 71 to 78 years of age, reported no significant difference of survival between patients less than 70 or greater than 71 years who underwent radical prostatectomy for localized disease. Caution should be used for older men who have organ confined prostate cancer to opt for surgery when other options are available to maintain a good quality of life. To set your mind at ease and to seek a second or third opinion, ask your doctor to interpret the Partin Tables or the Memorial Sloan-Kettering nomograms for a prediction of the course of disease based on increasing PSA values, staging of cancer, and increasing Gleason scores. Partin Tables are at www.prostatecancer.org/ and Sloan Kettering nomograms at www.mskcc.org/mskcc/html/10088.cfm will provide you with another opinion.

Knowing your prostate profile and by using Partin Tables "there is 95 a percent accuracy" according to Dr. Walsh, for the likelihood of having one of the following conditions: organ-confined disease, capsular penetration, cancer in the seminal vesicles or lymph nodes. Dr. Scardino was more cautious citing that the Sloan-Kettering nomogram as well as Partin Tables are not infallible and they are not intended to make decisions for you – there is a plus or minus 10 percent error built in. Several nomograms are cited in the literature for the progression of prostate cancer. Partin Tables are still widely used predictors of pathological stage in men with localized prostate cancer. Dr. Steuber and investigators stated that Partin Tables have limitations for men with transition zone prostate cancer. They noted that men with tumour characteristics of the transition zone for prostate cancer differ from those of the peripheral zone prostate cancer and those differences appear to undermine the accuracy of Partin Tables for predicting the accuracy of pathological stage. Men with T3a disease or if the cancer has extended beyond the capsule are not good candidates for surgery; external beam radiation and hormonal therapy may be recommended for this stage of cancer. However, for some men with minimal spread of cancer outside the prostate capsule or for transition zone cancer with a high PSA level, and with a Gleason score of less than 8, having surgery may be one possible option. Your urologist will of course advise if it is wise to proceed with surgery or radiation or both.

Cancer in the transition zone takes longer to escape the capsule even when a high PSA is reported. Dr. Walsh reported that "about 25 percent of these men turn out to have organ-confined disease." If there is recurrent disease after radical prostatectomy then external beam radiotherapy is a recommended option if the cancer has not spread beyond the prostate bed. If surgery is not the first option then the next best option for organ-confined disease, in my opinion, would be brachytherapy and perhaps followed by external beam radiation. What about the person with cancer that is not life-threatening and confined to his prostate but is older than 75 years? Watchful waiting or active surveillance could be a recommended option. If he is in poor health and with an estimated life expectancy of 10 years and his cancer is confined to the prostate, then objectified active surveillance could be recommended. An oncologist or urologist will provide the best advice for each patient's health profile. The advice provided in this and other chapters on diagnosis and treatment options are not meant to replace the recommendations of physicians.

Chapter 8

Incontinence, Erectile Dysfunction, Sexuality and Treatment Options

By reading this chapter you will learn:

- How does incontinence develop and its incidence after treatment.
- How to alleviate the symptoms of incontinence.
- What is erectile dysfunction?
- What should Canadians know about sexuality and erectile dysfunction?
- The incidence of erectile dysfunction after surgery or radiation.
- How is an erection initiated?
- How to treat erectile dysfunction to restore sexual potency.

Incontinence

Incontinence is the inability to hold urine in the bladder and this condition may be temporary following aggressive treatment for prostate cancer. Incontinence is infrequently a permanent side effect following surgery or radiation. Any damage to the external sphincter muscles will likely cause incontinence. There is a greater risk of a man experiencing extended incontinence following surgery than after radiation treatment. After surgery the patient is given a series of exercises to perform to strengthen his pelvic muscles in order to reduce incontinence. These Kegel exercises teach the patient to contract his muscles and hold them; it is like pulling everything "up inside" and not "pushing down." There are a variety of aids that are recommended to prevent any embarrassment of urine leakage when needed; these include the use of undergarment materials or pads to absorb any urine. You may expect to have incontinence lasting from a few days to weeks or even months following surgery or radiation. Do not be discouraged if incontinence continues longer. You have to be patient with this unfortunate condition. Make an appointment to see your urologist or oncologist if incontinence persists for longer than several weeks.

How is the male anatomy constructed for bladder control? Normally there are three separate structures that control urine flow from the bladder; the internal sphincter located at the neck of the bladder and adjacent to the prostate, the prostate gland itself, and the external sphincter muscle below the prostate gland. Only the external sphincter muscles are left intact after surgery (without complications), and they must be saved during the operation. As a man ages he loses the ability to use that muscle so men older than 70 years of age have more difficulty recovering from incontinence after surgery than younger males. Older men may opt to have 3-dimensional conformal radiation to reduce the incidence of incontinence instead of surgery. One test for continence is if you are dry before going to the toilet or after sitting and when you stand up and can hold the urge to go, then you are on the way to being continent. A study at Johns Hopkins reported that after surgery about 50 percent of men are wearing no pads at three months; 80 percent are wearing no pads at six months, and 90 to 93 percent of men are dry at twelve months. There is a small percent of men who remain incontinent for longer than one year. There is also a 98 percent chance that a man will be continent within 18 months to two years after surgery. Avoid drinking coffee, beer, tea and soft drinks if incontinence is a concern. Patients treated with external beam radiotherapy in one British Columbia study developed very low rates of incontinence – 4.7 percent occasionally used pads; 0.6 percent used pads intermittently, and 0.6 percent used incontinence pads regularly.

The Kegel isometric exercises (named after Dr. Arnold Kegel, a gynecologist) will help strengthen your sphincter muscles. Start your urine stream and after two to three seconds stop the stream by contracting your buttocks muscles. Tighten your buttocks and hold the flow back for about 5 seconds; repeat as many times as convenient. Do not over-practice this method throughout the day, but generally when you are passing urine and shortly thereafter. Be sure not to hold your breath when doing the Kegel exercises. Kegel exercises should not be performed while the catheter is in place. Wait for a few days after the catheter is removed before doing the exercises. Also, while not passing urine you should contract your pelvic floor muscles and hold the contraction for about ten seconds, relax for about five seconds; repeat ten times a day. Consult with your physician about these exercises and any precautions to follow. Men anticipating surgery should learn these exercises in advance. If after six months to one year there is little change in your incontinence condition, you should make an appointment with your urologist to discuss other options for treating the condition.

The plumbing system does not always work as efficiently after surgery or radiation; aging and the trauma of treatment weaken the external sphincter muscles. However, if the plumbing system still does not work and you continue to wear incontinence pads after 18 months to two years, then other options are available. Your urologist will guide you on which option to consider. The Bard Cunningham Clamp is made of soft rubber cushions and is sometimes used to control dribbling or small volume incontinence. Your urologist will first investigate your condition by doing a cystoscopic examination of the bladder neck and whether it is necessary to do a *collagen injection* (Figure 8.1). It takes several injections of collagen for the best results and the material may take about one month to set. Collagen tends to make the sphincter muscles more efficient. Not all men should have the collagen implants because some men are allergic to the material and if incontinence is severe it may not even work. If you have "urgency incontinence" (urine leaks out because you can't get to the toilet on time), then certain drugs of the anticholinergic medication type such as Benadryl may help. Other drugs such as Detrol, Ditropan, Sanctura, Enablex and Vesicare have been recommended to decrease urgency and frequency incontinence; those five drugs work by blocking the nerve impulses to the bladder that cause it to contract and leak. Ask your urologist, oncologist or your general practitioner which is the best drug for your condition and the possible side effects. The artificial sphincter implant is the last method for continued lengthy incontinence and it requires specialized surgery. Men should consider this treatment as a last resort because complications can arise from the invasive surgery.

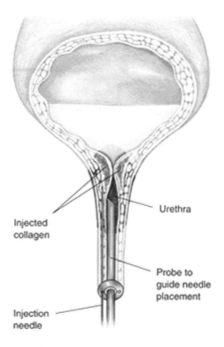

Figure 8.1: Collagen implant procedure. Adapted from the National Kidney and Urologic Diseases Information Clearinghouse, National Institute of Health.

Erectile Dysfunction and Restoring Potency

Erectile dysfunction or the inability to achieve and maintain an erection affects a high percent of men who have been treated for prostate cancer. Impotence or erectile dysfunction (ED) may be a temporary or permanent condition, depending on many factors including a preoperative potency or impotency, a man's age and health, whether one or two or no nerves are spared after surgery, or after being treated with external beam radiation, brachytherapy or hormonal therapy. *It is important to note that ED is not an inevitable result of aging.* The incidence of erectile dysfunction is also quite high after HIFU and Cryosurgery procedures. Most men are concerned about erectile dysfunction even before they have had any aggressive treatment. Normally, a man's ability to maintain an erection decreases as he ages. Many men experience ED without having been treated for prostate cancer. Men with health concerns such as diabetes, diseases of the blood vessels, after suffering a stroke, spinal cord injury, or those who have ingested certain drugs or alcohol can develop erectile dysfunction. Erectile dysfunction caused by overuse of alcohol and substance abuse can be reversed by abstaining from those products. Consult the *Male Health Centres* and the *Canadian Male Sex Health Council* websites listed below for additional information on the causes relating to ED.

A Massachusetts Male Aging Study survey of over 1 700 men aged 40 to 70 years reported that 52 percent of men had some degree of erectile dysfunction and almost 10 percent had complete erectile dysfunction. It is believed that about 2-3 million men in Canada suffer from ED. Testosterone levels slowly begin to decline starting at about age 40; about 20 percent of men report inadequate erections by age 50 and the problem increases as men age. By age 80, about 50 percent of healthy men are unable to achieve and maintain an erection. At age 60, about one-third of a man's testosterone level drops. Diabetes or other vascular problems such as hardening of the arteries impedes blood flow. Men over 50 years of age with health problems experience a 30 percent chance of ED than their healthy peers. A man with symptoms and conditions of erectile dysfunction may never regain his potency after treatment for prostate cancer. *Psychological factors* also play a role in the ability to maintain an erection. The psychological aspects of ED include relationship problems, depression, stress-related concerns such as financial problems, chronic pain, mental illness and performance anxiety. The latter is believed to release adrenaline which lowers the flow of blood to the penis. The following websites contain useful information about erectile dysfunction: www.malehealth.com, www.cmshc.org and www.impotence.org. The *Male Health Centres* and the *Canadian Male Sex Health Council* websites have developed an interest in men's health and particularly in sexual function. Dr. Richard Casey, the Director of the Male Health Centres in Ontario, may offer a second opinion to men and their spouses or partners, after consultation with their primary care physicians or specialists. For more information on how to contact Dr. Casey and his staff, call 905.338.3130 to speak to a receptionist; there is a fee for consultations with Dr. Casey. An interesting and recommended book, *Intimacy with Impotence* by Ralph Alterowitz and his wife Barbara, discusses erectile dysfunction, therapies and medications, and practical advice about lovemaking and more; it is a must read for couples dealing with intimacy issues.

As mentioned earlier, radical prostatectomy, radiation therapy, brachytherapy, hormonal therapy or castration can contribute significantly to the incidence of erectile dysfunction. Hormone therapy or castration as options for treating prostate cancer blocks testosterone level which is responsible in promoting a man's libido and the ability to achieve an erection. Even without hormonal therapy, the level of a man's testosterone keeps declining with age. Dr. Alvaro Morales at the Centre for Urological Research at Queens University in Ontario explained that low testosterone levels affect prostate health, cholesterol level, increase red blood cells, sleep deprivation and liver toxicity, to name a few effects. Dr. Morales advocates testosterone replacement therapy in men with no prostate problems but with low testosterone levels. Dr. Greenstein and investigators evaluated the efficacy of testosterone gel alone and the gel with sildenafil in hypogonadal (low levels of testosterone) patients with ED. Using both sildenafil and testosterone improved the effect on patients with ED more than taking testosterone alone. Male menopause or andropause is recognized as a normal part of aging due to androgen deficiency in some men; it is associated with an increasing decline in their sexuality, increased mental irritability, decreased muscle strength and decline in overall energy level.

Surgery, radiation therapy, brachytherapy, cryotherapy or high intensity focused ultrasound can damage the carvernous nerves which run alongside the prostate gland and to the penis and can result in erectile dysfunction. It may not be possible to save the neurovascular bundles during every surgery. Some surgeons will perform a *bilateral nerve graft* to replace the resected cavernous nerves. Dr. Kim and colleagues reported recovery of erectile function in men who underwent bilateral nerve graft during surgery when the cavernosal nerves could not be spared. The greatest return of potency in the men in this study was 14 to 18 months after surgery. The carvernous nerves and blood vessels are responsible for promoting erectile potency. There is a combination of chemical responses involved in achieving normal erections. The basic physiology for initiating an erection operates with the "mind-body" combination is a very complex process. The psychological sensation of pleasure is in the brain and the physiological actions involve the reproductive organs, muscles and the entire body. The sexual sensations may be simplified through the five senses of sight, touch, smell, hearing and taste. The brain then receives those sensations such as a "desire" for sex and then the "arousal" state ensues in both sexes. Testosterone, in addition to the brain, is also needed for arousal in the male. The cavernous nerves release nitric oxide which gives a signal to the penile blood vessels to allow the penis to receive more blood into the spongy erectile tissues. The result is an erection. As sexual stimulation intensifies, sperm and secretions from the prostate and seminal vesicles, collectively known as semen, are expelled from the penis in spurts by the contractions of muscles. Following a male orgasm and ejaculation, different neurotransmitters are released and the corporal tissues constrict to allow for the leakage of blood out of the penis that then assumes a flaccid state. After an ejaculation comes the refractory phase when further stimulation does not bring about an erection; older men experience a longer refractory period. A man's ejaculate may consist of up to 400 millions sperm cells and its volume is an average of 3-4 millilitres of semen in a healthy and younger male.

Following external beam radiation, about 25 to 50 percent of men develop erectile dysfunction, a lower incidence rate than with surgery. Many men who undergo radiotherapy initially lose their sexual potency for several months following treatment; sexual potency returns gradually. One chemical, endothelin -1, seems to increase after radiotherapy and it is responsible for constriction of localized blood vessels so there is less dilation or relaxation of blood vessels coming to the penis. Dr. Stacy Elliot at the University of British Columbia, and a member of the Canadian Male Sexual Health Council (www.cmshc.org), concludes it is important to control your sugar level to maintain normal sexual activity – an increase in sugar levels could cause an increase in ED. She also noted that smoking, high blood pressure and elevated cholesterol levels affect the endothelial tissues of the penis that need a ready supply of blood. By reducing any cardiovascular risk, ED will decrease. ED can also point to a silent heart condition.

What about the effects of post-operative surgery in relationship to the achievement of sexual potency? As mentioned earlier, the incidence rates of sexual dysfunction following surgery vary between individuals and from one surgeon to the next. Some men recover within months, others may take up to four years and some may never recover. Rates of sexual dysfunction following surgery vary from one study to the next and with the experience of the surgeon. Rates of sexual dysfunction range from as low as 18 percent to over 70 percent according to the literature. Many studies have documented the incidence of sexual dysfunction following surgery, external beam radiation and brachytherapy. One interesting study at the Stanford University School of Medicine reviewed 459 men of a mean age of 64 years after having radical prostatectomy. Erectile dysfunction was evaluated on those men before and after their surgery. *Erectile dysfunction* is defined as the persistent incapability to achieve erection and/or maintain an erection strong enough to have vaginal penetration. All patients in the Stanford study were assessed at T1a to T2c staging except for two men. Of the total number of men studied, only 51 or 11 percent remained sexually potent one year after their surgery. When one nerve was spared the potency success rate was 13.3 percent; when two nerves were spared the potency success rate was 31.9 percent. When no nerves were spared the potency rate was a mere 1.1 percent. In summary, the recovery rate was low.

In a *JAMA* study, Dr. Janet Stanford and investigators reported on the incidence of urinary and sexual function after radical prostatectomy for localized prostate cancer. In that survey, a total of 1 291 black, white and Hispanic men aged 39 to 79 years. The recovery rates after 18 or more months following surgery were noted. In total, 8.4 percent of men remained incontinent and 60 percent of men remained impotent. Among those men who were potent before surgery, erectile dysfunction (ED) with non-nerve sparing following surgery was 65.6 percent; with unilateral nerve-sparing the incidence of ED was 59 percent, and with bilateral nerve-sparing it was 56 percent. The survey suggests that "radical prostatectomy is associated with significant erection dysfunction and some decline in urinary function." When the neurovascular bundles are spared, the potency rate improves. Another significant survey was conducted by Dr. Kundu and colleagues on sexual potency and continence on a large population of 3 477 men who had radical prostatectomy performed by urologist William Catalona. Dr. Catalona is a well-known urology surgeon in the United States. Excluded from the findings were men who were not reliably potent before surgery and those who did not undergo nerve-sparing. The study provided evidence that "erections sufficient for intercourse occurred in 76% of preoperatively potent men treated with bilateral sparing and 53% of men with unilateral or partial nerve sparing surgery." Recovery of potency and incontinence was more common in younger men within 18 months of surgery. The recovery from urinary incontinence occurred in 93 percent of men. These findings indicated that nerve-sparing surgery can be performed with favourable potency being restored after 18 months and with urinary continence success. According to the study, better results are achieved in younger patients and those who were potent before surgery while complications in surgery are minimized with the experience of the surgeon.

The Stanford University study, Dr. Janet Stanford's study, and the large cohort of 3 447 men in the study conducted by Dr. Kundu and others, with Dr. Catalona as the performing surgeon, demonstrated that sexual potency after radical prostatectomy was related to the number of neurovascular bundles spared, potency or frequency of intercourse preoperatively and patient age. In my opinion, the above studies were comprehensive and meaningful for post-operative impotence and incontinence considerations as well as for counselling of men before and after having surgery or other aggressive treatment for prostate. Regaining sexual potency is not an overnight event but may take two years or longer. Delayed recovery of nerve action may be due to stretching of the nerves during surgery or injury in attempts to control bleeding as well as the effects of surgical trauma. Dr. Arthur Burnett, in a recent report in *JAMA*, noted that the cavernous nerves are functionally inactive for as long as two years after surgery even when the nerve-sparing operation is successful. A very high percentage of men who did not have nerve-sparing surgery in all the studies cited remained sexually dysfunctional. Older men may never regain sexual potency and especially those who did not have adequate erectile function before their surgery or radiotherapy even when both nerves are spared. The good news is that after one year or more, many men regain their sexual potency after nerve-sparing surgery and a high percent of them remain continent.

Sexuality: A Canadian Study

Drs. Auld and Brock are members of the Canadian Male Sexual health Council and reported their findings in the *Journal of Sexual and Reproductive Medicine*. They documented interviews with over 3 000 men and women from the Atlantic Canada across to British Columbia on sexuality and erectile dysfunction. Of the men and women who were interviewed, 75 percent were involved in a relationship and 80 percent lived with their partners at the time. The average number of sexual partners in their history was six but men reported having more sexual partners in their lifetime. Older men were less likely to discuss issues of sexuality than younger men. Sexual performance and infidelity were the most difficult subjects to discuss. About 93 percent of men and 91 percent of women considered sex an important part of their lives. However, about 80 percent of the men and women had not discussed issues such as ED and sexuality with their physicians. Because most of the men had not discussed issues of ED with their partners, their partners felt their partners were having sexual relations with someone else.

Respondents to the survey answered that ED was mostly due to psychological factors rather than existing physical conditions. In the Canadian survey, 90 percent of respondents felt that their partners "were understanding" about ED, but 38 percent said that ED had put a strain on their relationship. About 88 percent agreed that ED is a medical condition but only 25 percent of men with ED felt that it was easy to discuss the topic with a physician. Another article in the *Journal of Sexual Reproductive Medicine* outlined a "Position Statement" on sexuality education, and counseling guidelines for primary care physicians. It concludes that sexuality should be introduced to a child in gradual, age-appropriate manner. Physicians can be helpful in providing information and support to parents in this regard. It is also important for physicians and other professionals to learn about aspects of sexuality development. Physicians should ask their patients about their sexual health and encourage them to discuss similar matters with their spouses or partners. The Levitra website at www.levitra.com has a Sexual Health Checklist that can help a patient initiate a discussion on erectile function with his doctor – click on "Talking to Your Doctor." At the American Cancer Society website, (www.cancer.org) it includes a section titled Additional Resources and lists a recommended text: *Sexuality and Cancer: For the Man who has Cancer and his Partner.*

Treating Erectile Dysfunction with Modern Medicine

The penis is an important anatomical structure comprising mainly of blood vessels, nerves, and smooth muscle tissues. The arterial supply to the corpora cavernosa or spongy tissues of the penis is composed mainly of three branches of the common penile artery – the cavernosal arteries, dorsal penile artery and the bulbourethral artery. The cavernosal arteries carry blood to the erectile tissues while the dorsal artery is mainly respon-

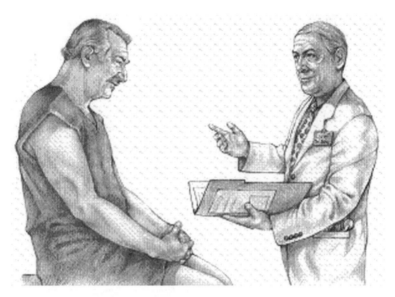

Figure 8.2: Talking with your doctor about ED as a medical problem. Illustration adapted from the National Institute of Diabetes and Digestive and Kidney Diseases, National Institute of Health.

sible for engorgement of the glans penis. Arteries provide the blood to the corpora cavernosa when the muscles relax while drainage of blood from the veins is blocked. A smaller chamber or the corpus spongiosum surrounds the urethra also becomes filled with blood that is supplied to the glans or tip of the penis. The glans penis is normally covered by the foreskin; sometimes the foreskin is surgically removed right after birth in a procedure called circumcision. The main erectile tissues are the two corpora cavernosa bodies on the shaft of the penis. The spongy tissues consist of microscopic chambers called sinuses. It is worth noting that after radical prostatectomy the penis is known to reduce in length or becomes slightly retracted. A study conducted by Dr. Munding and colleagues in Tucson, Arizona, found that 71 percent of the 31 patients had a decrease of penile length that ranged from 0.5 cm to 4.0 cm at three months after radical prostatectomy. Dr. Savoie and investigators at the University of Miami School of Medicine support the findings that penile length after radical prostatectomy is reduced. The study included 124 men who consented to penile measurements before surgery and repeat measurements during three-month intervals.

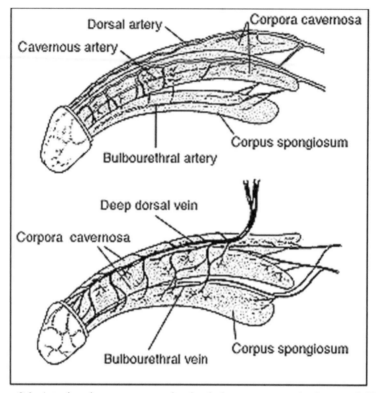

Figure 8.3: Arteries shown at top and veins below penetrate the long and filled cavities running the penis. Nerves run alongside the dorsal artery are not shown. Adapted from the National Kidney and Urologic Diseases Information Clearinghouse, National Institute of Health.

Since the emergence of Viagra (sildenafil), Cialis (tadalafil) and Levitra (vardenafil), drug companies through their advertising have educated the public about the chemical ingredients of these drugs and provided warnings about possible side effects. A few guidelines on these drugs can be summarized as follows: Viagra has a 4-5 hour half-life and should be taken about one hour before use, preferably on an empty stomach or about two hours after a fatty meal. Levitra has a 4-5 hour half-life and it may be taken with a low fat meal one hour before expected relations; and Cialis has a half-life of about 18 hours and up to 36 hours with no food restrictions. A study conducted by Dr. Hatzichristou and colleagues in Europe found that tadalafil may provide men with ED more flexibility in deciding when to attempt sexual intercourse and it had a higher intercourse success rate through 36 hours after dose compared with the placebo group.

It is important to know about nitric oxide and its effects before discussing the modern drugs for treating ED. When a man is sexually aroused, a natural body substance known as nitric oxide is released by nerve endings in the penis, initiating relaxation of the smooth muscles. The penis receives nerves from both the autonomic and somatic pathways. By definition, the autonomic nerve has control over internal organs such as increasing or decreasing heart rate; the somatic nerves generally control muscle activity. One branch of the autonomic system is referred to as the parasympathetic nerve that brings about relaxation within the penis, resulting in the engorgement of the corpora cavernosa and corpus spongiosum. Those tissues, when relaxed, cause the smooth muscles to become dilated or expand. Arteries and veins both add blood to the penis when it is dilating; when the veins become stretched, the penis begins to elongate. The spongy mass is filled with blood and as tissues in the penis continue to expand, blood is prevented from leaving the penis. The spongy chambers finally become engorged with blood during sexual stimulation and activity. Nitric oxide is important in starting the physiological process from the nerve endings to the corpus cavernosa tissues in the penis in the birth of an erection. Without the action of the brain and neurotransmitters for initiating the desire to have sexual intercourse, the arousal state may not be initiated and drugs like Viagra may not work.

How does a drug like **Viagra** or its chemical ingredient **sildenafil** work to improve sexual potency? The physiological-neural event to initiate an erection with drugs like sildenafil is a relatively new science. First, neurotransmitters release nitric oxide in the corpus cavernosum with the resulting increase of a chemical called cyclic guanosine monophosphate, or cGMP as it is abbreviated. The cGMP promotes dilation of smooth muscles within the penis and increases the flow of blood. During sexual arousal the autonomic nerve impulses elevate cGMP in smooth muscle cells and the erectile tissues become filled with blood. There is an important natural "off switch" discovered for cGMP; it is an enzyme known as *phosphodiesterase5* (PDE5). PDE5 is responsible for degradation of cGMP in the corpus cavernosum. Sildenafil, tadalafil and vardenafil are known to *inhibit* the phosphodiesterase5 enzyme or the "off switch"

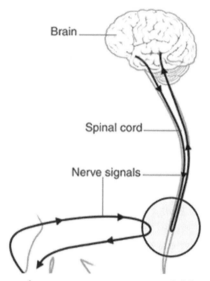

Figure 8.4: Motor and sensory nerves operate to initiate an erection. Adapted from the National Institute of Diabetes and Digestive and Kidney Diseases, National Institute of Health.

allowing for a ready supply of cGMP. There are eleven known variations of phosphodiesterases that have their effect on other parts of the body but PDE5 has its specific effect on the penis. The three modern drugs mentioned block one form of phosphodiesterase to the penis. Thus when phosphodiesterase5 is blocked, it will allow for a continuous supply of cGMP and the neurotransmitters to continue to function for the release of nitric oxide. The physiological phenomenon that ensues is dilation of smooth muscles allowing blood to enter freely into the penis that becomes trapped in the corpora tissues, resulting in an erection. Sildenafil, tadalafil, and vardenafil act as phosphodiesterase5 inhibitors to keep the cGMP switch turned on to initiate and maintain an erection. After sexual arousal or excitement, orgasm and ejaculation, a man's penis and mental state enter a refractory phase and second erection cannot be initiated during that period.

Cialis works faster and its effect lasts longer than Viagra or Levitra but it applies the same physiological principle. However, those drugs will not cause an erection unless the man is sexually aroused; the brain (Figure 8.4) has to be involved for nerves and medication to work. Sex is indeed a mind-body phenomenon. It is important to ask about the side effects of these drugs and to be aware of the consequences of overuse. Your doctor and pharmacist should inform you of the danger of taking this medication in conjunction with other drugs such as nitroglycerin and alpha blockers. It is estimated that more than 33 million men in Canada and in the United States suffer from erectile dysfunction. Dr. Goldstein and colleagues carried out a 24-week dose-response study on 532 men who experienced erectile dysfunction with sildenafil (at 25, 50 or 100 mg doses) and a placebo. Increasing doses of sildenafil (Viagra) were associated with improved sexual potency. During the last four weeks of treatment in the dose-escalation study, 69 percent of all attempts at sexual intercourse were successful for men taking sildenafil compared with 22 percent of those on the placebo.

The drug **tadalafil**, sold under the name of **Cialis,** was tested in a double blind study by Dr. Seftel in the U.S. and Puerto Rico on 207 men with mild to severe erectile dysfunction and reported in *The Journal of Urology.* The men in the survey were not treated for prostate cancer. Over the course of 12 weeks, 20 milligrams of tadalafil or Cialis was given to the experimental group (non-placebo) and the placebo group received none. The result was a significant improvement of erectile function – 82 percent of the men taking tadalafil versus 20 percent in the placebo group had improved erections. The study reported that the most successful intercourse attempts occurred between 4 and 36 hours after taking tadalafil. Cialis was well tolerated by participants in the study and may be taken without food restrictions. In another study reported by Dr. Brock and colleagues in *The Journal of Urology,* **vardenafil**, sold as **Levitra,** another *phosphodiesterase inhibitor,* was administered in a double blind study on 440 men with erectile dysfunction for a duration of 12 weeks. Two different doses of 10 and 20 mg of vardenafil were given and the placebo group received none. Among men with bilateral nerve bundle-sparing surgery after radical prostatectomy who were taking 20 mg vardenafil, the degree of sexual potency restored was 71 percent while 60 percent of men taking 10 mg of the drug had their potency restored. About 12 percent in the placebo group (not taking vardenafil) had their sexual potency restored. The conclusion was that "in men with severe ED after nerve sparing radical retropubic prostatectomy, vardenafil significantly improved key indices of erectile function."

"In the Johns Hopkins experience of men who are unable to have sexual intercourse more than one year after an operation in which both neurovascular bundles were spared, 80 percent are able to have successful intercourse after treatment with Viagra" according to Dr. Walsh in his research. If you have an irregular heartbeat, have low or high blood pressure symptoms or retina pigmentosa, Viagra, Cialis and Levitra are not for you. Men who take nitroglycerin for angina should not be taking these drugs. Remember, these drugs do not work if you are not sexually aroused. There are mild side effects with Viagra, Cialis, or Levitra; it is important to read the information that is provided with the drug and to ask the pharmacist to provide you with any information about drug interactions. An initial dose of 50 milligrams of Viagra taken one hour before sexual activity is generally recommended; some men may only need 25 milligrams while others may need to take up to 100 milligrams of Viagra. Talk to your doctor if this dose does not work for you. Also discuss this medication with your spouse or partner. I am sure that in the future more effective drugs for treating erectile dysfunction with fewer side effects will emerge. In the August 2005 issue of *Insights Newsletter* of the Prostate Cancer Research Institute, Dr. Auerbach listed six new medications that are being tested that showed promise for treating ED, including medications with similar PDE5 inhibitors of the drugs described above. The following websites provide information on these drugs, ED and sexual health matters: www.cialis.com/index.jsp, www.levitra.com, and www.viagra.ca.

Loss of nocturnal erections after nerve-sparing surgery may be a "detriment to recovery of erectile function. Nocturnal erections provide a means by which oxygenated blood routinely bathes the corporal tissues..." according to Dr. Carter's letter in a *Johns Hopkins Bulletin*. He contends that a total absence of erections lead to damage or scarring of the corporal tissues due to a lack of oxygen. In a double blind study of 76 men with normal preoperative erectile function, the men were prescribed Viagra at night for nine months after surgery to determine if sexual potency could improve or be restored. Men were given either 50 or 100 milligrams of Viagra and a third group received the placebo. The finding showed that 27 percent of men receiving Viagra had spontaneous erectile function compared with 4 percent in the placebo group. The efficacy of Viagra or sildenafil may be due to improved oxygenation of the penile tissue. The study was never published and you should be wary of daily use of Viagra after surgery. In a sample population of 53 men studied by Dr. Matthew and colleagues, 80 percent who had bilateral nerve-sparing surgery after radical prostatectomy reported positive responses with sildenafil while of the men who had no nerves spared none reported positive responses with sildenafil. Neurotransmitters must be intact if these modern drugs are to be effective.

Well before the availability of Viagra, 70 percent of men who had nerve-sparing surgery in one Johns Hopkins study had return of erections within one year. Did Viagra have the desired effect or did the men gradually have their erection restored without taking Viagra? That question still remains unanswered. In a Cross-National Survey on Men's Health Issues, a population based international survey correlating patient age and overall health with the prevalence of ED was studied. Dr. Shabsigh and investigators in that study used a cohort of 28 691 men age 20 to 75 years who completed a screening questionnaire. Respondents in the oldest age group of 70 to 75 years experienced a 14-fold higher risk in ED than respondents in the 20 to 29 year age group. They found that ED was positively associated with poor overall health, including prostate and urinary problems. They also noted that the presence of ED should alert physicians to the likelihood of common comorbidities such as hypertension and diabetes.

What about taking testosterone supplements? As mentioned above, there may be a need to provide *hormone replacement therapy* for some men with hypogonadal (low testosterone) conditions and ED. Some men believe that taking testosterone supplements will restore their sexual potency. Men should use extreme caution with testosterone supplementation for lack of libido or erectile dysfunction. One note of caution for men who still have healthy prostates: prostate cancer may become "clinically apparent within months to a few years after the initiation of testosterone treatment" according to research done by Dr. Gaylis and investigators. Dr. J. Kellog Parsons and colleagues evaluated serum androgen concentrations and prostate cancer risk. The results from a study of 794 members of the Baltimore Longitudinal Study of Aging found that free testosterone was associated with an increased age-adjusted risk of prostate cancer. One study conducted by Dr. Severi and others reported that "some recent studies have even suggested that high testosterone levels might be protective particularly against aggressive cancer." Testosterone replacement therapy should be reserved for men with abnormally low testosterone levels and only on the advice of his physician. Men receiving testosterone therapy should be regularly monitored for prostate cancer. Dr. Casey noted that "7% of men aged 40 to 50 years, 20% of men aged 60 to 80 years, and 35% over 80 years of age have below- normal serum testosterone." He stated that depression was a common clinical condition producing decreased libido in men of all ages. Depressed men with low libido may benefit from testosterone administration. Dr. Casey also said that in hypogonadal men, administration of testosterone increases muscle and bone metabolism and an improvement in their quality of life.

Other Methods of Treating ED

As mentioned above, a high percentage of younger men and those who were potent before any aggressive treatment have their potency restored if the nerves were spared or not damaged. In addition to using modern drugs for treating ED, there are other options available for a man who experiences erectile dysfunction. It is still possible for a man to achieve an erection and continue to have sexual intercourse even if he suffers from ED. I was pleasantly surprised to listen to men openly discussing their personal problems at some of the meetings of the Vancouver Prostate Support and Awareness Group (PSA) of which I was the editor of the *PSA Newsletter* some years ago; it could be one source of information for men who wish to openly discuss ED and possible ways to treat it. Men and spouses or partners should also receive *sexual therapy* by professionals as a means of identifying sexual problems and recommended treatment options. Since many younger men have to cope with sexual dysfunction after surgery or radiation, urologists and oncologists should be taught to offer sexual dysfunction counselling to men and their spouses or partners.

The urologist may prescribe a bi-mixture or tri-mixture of alprostadil, phentolamine and papaverine for **penile self-injections** but few men reportedly seem satisfied with this treatment option because they do not like the idea of having to administer injections into their own penises. The success rate for achieving an erection with this method is 80 to 90 percent successful. It is important to follow instructions from your urologist. Be sure not to self-administer more than the prescribed amount of this drug as complications may develop. Prolonged erection or priapism sometimes occurs when higher concentrations are administered. If the condition of priapism persists, and prolonged pain ensues, it may be necessary to have minor surgery to drain blood from the penis. The mixture of drugs has to be refrigerated or it will lose its effectiveness. It usually takes about five minutes to achieve an erection with a penile injection. Your urologist should fully explain the effects of this medication and the injection process. Be warned that many men suffer painful erections after administering Alprostadil or prostaglandin E1, mainly after having surgery but less so after radiotherapy.

There is a **topical vasodilator ointment** that contains a derivative of Alprostadil, and sold as a product known as **Befar**, which is applied to the glans or tip of the penis. In one trial, 83 percent of men with erectile dysfunction were satisfied with Befar. In a trial at Peking University People's Hospital in Beijing, Dr. Jiang and investigators reported that after taking the synthetic PGE1 cream in a placebo controlled study, 63 percent of the men using the cream showed significant improvement in potency as against 10 percent in the placebo group. Common side effects with Befar include mild pain of the penis and urethra. Befar acts as a vasodilator (widening of blood vessels) and treatment is less invasive. Befar is a product from Hong Kong and men should talk to their urologists before using it. An herbal medicine that needs investigating is **Korean red ginseng.** A double blind study was conducted on the efficacy of Korean red ginseng on 45 patients with clinically diagnosed erectile dysfunction. The ginseng dose was 900 mg taken three times daily. "Function scores were significantly higher in patients treated with Korean red ginseng than those who received the placebo…60 percent of the patients answered that Korean red ginseng improved erection" according to Dr. Hong and others. The data show that Korean red ginseng can be an effective alternative for treating male erectile dysfunction. On the subject of herbal medicine, Dr. Fleshner and colleagues in Canada investigated seven herbal products and their ingredients that can be obtained through the internet and at health food stores. They found that a significant number of natural products sold for treating ED contained phosphodiesterase5 inhibitors (PDE5), the active ingredient found in modern prescription drugs. Those so-called natural products can be potentially dangerous since the customer is unaware of the presence of PDE5 and the danger of drug interactions. Consumers should be made more aware of the chemical composition in herbal products since the chemical ingredients are seldom known or revealed to the public. One website of interest as a guide to the efficacy of certain products claiming cures and informing the public of health-related frauds is www.quackwatch.org.

The Medicated Urethral System for Erection, or **MUSE**, is another method used for treating ED. A tiny suppository containing the synthetic form of prostaglandin E1 or Alprostadil is inserted into the urethra. It is easy to administer and you do not have to worry about injections. The suppository has to be inserted while standing and then the penis has to be massaged for about ten minutes for the drug to be absorbed into the smooth muscles. The one drawback is that this drug may cause a burning sensation and severe pain in the penis of men who had radical prostatectomy. MUSE works on about 40 to 55 percent of patients and is not effective with long-standing ED patients. MUSE seems to work better for men after having radiation therapy and for any man who developed erectile dysfunction without having any previous treatment for prostate cancer.

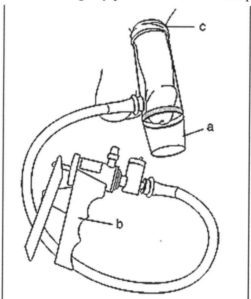

Figure 8.5: The vacuum-constrictor device and components: (a) plastic cylinder; (b) a hand pump; (c) elastic constricting ring. Adapted from the National Kidney and Urologic Diseases Clearinghouse, National Institute of Health.

The vacuum erection device uses a cylinder and a hand-held or automatic pump that creates a vacuum within a plastic tube; the flaccid penis is placed within the cylinder and becomes filled with blood in a vacuum environment, creating an artificial erection. A rubber ring or constricting ring is fitted at the base of the penis soon after achieving an erection to maintain its rigidity. One drawback is that the temperature of a man's penis may be cooler than when a normal erection is achieved. Your spouse or partner should be aware of any device or method you decide to use for regaining sexual potency. You should be taught how to use this device. Some companies sell devices and offer a 90 - day money back guarantee and the cost may go as high as $500.00 per unit. Cheaper units are just as effective so do your research before purchasing. Your urologist may have these devices in the office and can advise you on their use. The success rate with the vacuum device is about 80 percent satisfaction for achieving an erection.

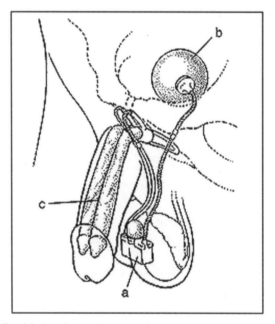

Figure 8.6: Inflatable implant with (a) pump in the scrotum; (b) fluid flows from this reservoir to two cylinders (c) in the penis. The cylinders expand to create an erection. Adapted from the National Kidney and Urologic Diseases Information Clearinghouse, National Institute of Health.

The bark from the evergreen yohimbehe tree in Africa produces the drug yohimbine but it is seldom prescribed; the results from this natural aphrodisiac are not satisfactory for most men. There are also some mild to severe side effects with using yohimbine. Finally, the penile implant or prosthesis is a semi-rigid or an inflatable device. Implants are invasive and require anesthesia and specialized surgery. Mechanical failure is possible and an additional operation may be necessary to repair the pump. The procedure is permanent and irreversible. Men and their spouses or partners should seek special counseling before considering this method for restoring ED; it is a treatment of last resort.

Summary

Regarding erectile dysfunction (ED) and incontinence after radical prostatectomy or radiation for clinically localized prostate cancer, it has been well documented that younger men recover faster than older men from incontinence and ED. For men with any comorbidities, such as vascular conditions, even without being treated for prostate cancer, the incidence of ED will probably increase, indicating that ED can be a prognostic health marker in men. ED may last for up to two years following aggressive treatment for prostate cancer. Dr. Burnett reported that when nerve-sparing surgery is accomplished after radical prostatectomy "between 65% and 85% of men eventually recover erectile dysfunction....but early recovery of natural erectile function is uncommon." Research in men recovering from post-radical prostatectomy indicates that 25 to 75 percent of them experience sexual dysfunction. "Approximately 60 percent of patients experience emotional distress related to their sexual dysfunction that may progress to long-term maladjustment in their relationships with their partners," according to by Dr. Matthew and others in a Journal of Urology article. Dr. O'Leary and others in their study of men with ED reported that sildenafil or Viagra produced "substantial improvements in self-esteem, confidence and relationship satisfaction" when compared with the placebo group.

Surgeon experience and the extent of a man's cancer determine whether the neurovascular bundles can be spared. The research conducted and discussed previously on erectile dysfunction should be a concern to men before pursuing aggressive treatment such as radical prostatectomy. The first priority is to eradicate your cancer; secondly, it is important for the surgeon to save the external sphincter muscles below the prostate gland, and thirdly, if possible, try to save the neurovascular bundles for restoring sexual potency. You are reminded that the information on treatment options presented in this chapter and throughout this book is not intended to replace the advice of your physician and trained health care professionals. The opinions expressed are my personal views and from the updated research cited in the literature. Consult your general practitioner, oncologists and urologists for expert advice. It is most important to initiate the discussion of sexual matters with your spouse or partner when both of you visit your doctor.

Chapter 9
Radiation Therapy and Additional Treatment Options

By reading this chapter you will learn:

- How does external beam radiation work and who should be treated?
- Conventional, three-dimensional and intensity modulated radiotherapy.
- What are the advantages of having external beam radiation with advanced technological systems?
- What are the side effects of external beam radiation?
- Who is eligible for seed implantation or brachytherapy?
- Brachytherapy with adjuvant external beam radiation.
- What are the side effects of brachytherapy?
- Androgen deprivation as neo-adjuvant and adjuvant therapy.
- Is there any advantage of intermittent androgen suppression?
- Chemotherapy and treatment recommendations for distant metastasis.
- Objectified active surveillance, its importance and who should be monitored.
- When cancer returns, what should be done?
- The ProstaScint scan and its importance.

External Beam Radiation Therapy

If surgery is not the best treatment option, then a combination of one or more of the following alternatives can be recommended by specialists: **external beam radiation therapy, brachytherapy, hormone therapy** or **objectified active surveillance.** Both cryotherapy and high intensity focused ultrasound have not been conclusively proven as conventional therapies yet. External beam radiation and brachytherapy are potential curative treatment options aside from radical prostatectomy. When radical prostatectomy is not possible due to extracapsular penetration or other factors such as a person's health, external beam radiation may be the most effective treatment option available. The patient's grade of cancer, PSA value and velocity, his age, cancer volume, staging of disease, and state of health should be known before any evaluation or decision for treatment with either external beam radiation or brachytherapy is considered. External beam radiation therapy is meant to direct high energy X-rays on the prostate gland and surrounding areas. The amount of radiation is measured in Gray (Gy) units, named after the famous English radiobiologist Louis Gray. The dose of radiation varies from 70 Gy to about 81 Gy per treatment based on the advice of the attending radiation oncologist. The patient should be informed of all options of treatment available for his age and his present state of health. If the cancer has advanced and has left the capsule of the prostate gland but is confined to the pelvic bed after radical prostatectomy, then radiotherapy is often deemed successful in alleviating symptoms, suppressing and killing cancer cells leading to a cure of prostate cancer. When there is a high risk of cancer spreading to the lymph nodes, these areas in the pelvic region may be treated with external beam radiation. Hormone therapy may be taken along with radiotherapy to provide a delay of cancer progression.

A Gleason score, Gleason grade, free PSA percent, cancer stage, tumour volume, total PSA value, PSA doubling time, and velocity are significant determining factors of any disease progression and the kind of treatment that is required. A PSA velocity of 0.5 to 0.75 within one year is cause for concern. With a rise in detectable PSA (greater than 10) or a doubling of PSA within six months to a year, and a Gleason score of 8 or higher, it is likely that cancer has invaded the lymph nodes and likely gone beyond the pelvic region. In *The Journal of Urology,* Dr. Cadeddu and colleagues cautioned that with a Gleason score of 8-10, with positive lymph nodes or positive seminal vesicles, no patient responded favourably to radiation therapy. Radiation oncologist Tyldesley at the Vancouver Cancer Clinic stated that the patient with this condition who received hormonal therapy for 2-3 years in addition to receiving radiation therapy increase the chance of cure and improved survival rates compared with radiation therapy alone for high risk patients. A man older than 70 years of age (with other health concerns and unable to tolerate hormonal therapy) may elect to have an orchiectomy followed by external beam radiation. Orchiectomy or castration deprives the prostate of testosterone which is an effective form of androgen deprivation without taking any anti-androgen drugs. Of course, the idea of having testicles removed is often associated with the end of a man's sexual life but he has to consider his survival time, the extent of his cancer and his quality of life when making any decision on his treatment. He must weigh the option of either taking hormonal therapy or having an orchiectomy that leaves a man permanently deprived of testosterone. A man whose life-expectancy is less than 10 years may be advised to have an orchiectomy. The radiation oncologist or urologist will advise and guide the patient on the best options based on the patient's health.

After an appointment with a radiation oncologist, the patient is given specific procedures to follow before radiation treatment begins. Health care providers use measurements from scans and calculations to determine the precise location at which to aim the beams of radiation. Small tattoos are marked on the patient's skin for directing the radiation during the treatment period. Treatment with external beam radiation may last from six to eight weeks and is done on an outpatient basis. Each treatment lasts only a few minutes each day and is usually done five days each week. Radiation is given by highly trained and skilled technologists and extreme procedural caution is followed. Patients may spend 30 to 40 minutes at the treatment centre and are free to return home. Most of the time at the clinic is spent preparing the patient for the radiation. The patient is immobilized to minimize movement during the dosing sessions. He may lie on his back with his knees slightly flexed or face down, depending on the oncologist and the patient's condition. The patient's target organ and anatomy are mapped by computer using a CT scan before the treatment. During treatment, the prostate is specifically targeted as structures shift from day to day and the immobilization of the patient has to be repeated. The treatment itself takes just a few minutes and is painless. Most patients are able to drive home while some men prefer to have others do the driving after treatment.

Treatment with external beam radiation is planned so as to minimize the risks of any side effects. The purpose of radiation therapy is to control the spread of cancer growth and to kill cancer cells. Cancer cells are "stunned" with the high energy X-rays by damaging the chromosomes; cancer cells are killed and any new growth is suppressed by radiation. Radiation is also known to induce programmed cell death or apoptosis, effectively causing cells to commit suicide. Since the radiation must pass through healthy tissues, some of those healthy cells are damaged as well. Successful radiation therapy depends on delivering the radiation in the most effective way and with the right dose as expressed in Grays. With standard radiation dosing, the patient may experience temporary skin irritation, nausea, fatigue, loss of appetite, loose stools or diarrhea, intestinal cramps, severe flatulence, irritation of the bladder, bowel urgency, rectal bleeding, rectal pain during the course of radiation treatment and following treatment. Any severe problems resulting from radiation should be reported to your radiation oncologist. Many of the effects from radiation therapy subside within weeks and months after treatment and are not permanent. Suppositories and medication are prescribed by your oncologist to reduce rectal inflammation or proctitis. During the course of treatment, health care professionals will inform you of what you should take or do to reduce any of the effects of radiation. After the therapy sessions are completed the patient will visit his oncologist for periodic follow-up examinations and tests.

A three-dimensional conformal radiotherapy (3DCRT) procedure developed in the late 1980s targets the cancer sites and reduces the radiation effects on adjacent tissues such as the rectum and bladder. Fewer side effects are experienced by patients using this more effective form of radiation therapy as compared with conventional radiation. The 3DCRT is now used extensively in Canada. The radiation oncologist uses a computer to shape the beams to the tumours with 3DCRT. Multiple X-ray beams are positioned using high-tech computers and aided by CT scan or MRI that measure the specific target region and delivers high doses of radiation. A very small number of men experience incontinence and the incidence is generally lower than with surgery. About 25 to 50 percent of men become impotent due to the scarring in the pelvic area and damage to the neurovascular bundles alongside the prostate gland. A study conducted by Dr. Liu and colleagues at the B.C. Cancer Agency on the incidence of urinary incontinence after external beam radiation reported very low incidence rates among patients. Most patients, however, respond well without any serious problems through this technological advancement of three-dimensional radiotherapy. There are fewer problems such as bleeding from the rectum and bladder irritation from 3DCRT than with the older conventional therapy. Radiation oncologists provide the optimum amount of radiation or Gy for the patient. The goal is to find the optimal radiation dose to kill all of the prostate cancer cells.

Oncologists often put patients on androgen deprivation before, during and after radiation therapy. The B.C. Cancer Agency recently announced the evaluation of the first of its kind three-dimensional ultrasound guidance system to determine its accuracy for pinpointing the prostate gland location during radiation therapy. A man's prostate gland can shift in his body from hour to hour and it can change its shape and size during the course of the therapy. Having this added dimension defined will reduce the risk of side effects as the prostate gland needs to be specifically targeted. The findings from this planned study by Dr. Berthelet on Vancouver

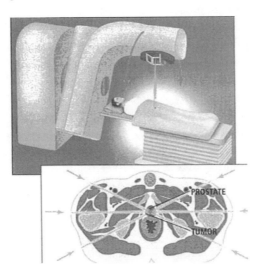

Figure 9.1: External Beam Radiation and three-dimensional beams targeted to the prostate gland. With permission from AstraZeneca Canada.

Island will be announced at a later date. Alternatively, the patient may be offered gold fiducial markers which are inserted into the prostate to accurately determine the position and target the prostate for treatment especially when high doses of greater than 74 Gy are used. When the study with ultrasound guidance is completed, oncologists will be able to compare this method with fiducial gold markers that are presently being used. Patients are also advised to have full bladders and to empty their bowels before dosing to minimize movement of the prostate gland. Radiation oncologist Tyldesley said that cure rates with 3DCRT are comparable to surgery and brachytherapy and there is some evidence that higher doses of radiation (78 Gy) may be more effective for some patients.

The *intensity modulated radiation therapy,* or IMRT procedure is another form of radiotherapy that uses many thinner beams of radiation to precisely target the prostate and spare other areas from the damaging effects of radiation. IMRT is an evolution from the 3DCRT using sophisticated computerized technology and is the most recent advance in the delivery of radiation. It sets a precise dose of radiation for the tumour or target volume while restricting the amounts of radiation to other tissues such as the rectum and bladder wall. In fact, IMRT may allow for higher doses of radiation to the prostate and target features. The target is hit from a number of directions with sub-beams of radiation while varying the intensity of doses. IMRT is available in Canada at the time of writing and shows promise of being used for treating prostate cancer. However, there is no proof to date that IMRT provides better outcome than 3DCRT for treating prostate cancer. IMRT is able to direct the radiation to the prostate while radiation to the rectum and other structures are minimized. "The incidence of bowel injuries, especially the serious ones, has been greatly reduced to 17 percent with 3D-Conformal radiation whereas the incidence with IMRT it was only 2 to 3 percent," according to Dr. Scardino's experience at the Memorial Sloan-Kettering Center. Only a small number of patients develop proctitis or radiation burn of the rectum with IMRT as compared with 3-D conformal therapy when very high doses of radiation are used. It remains unclear if any patients benefit from very high doses of radiation. Erectile dysfunction after IMRT and 3DCRT treatment is similar to brachytherapy and possibly superior to radical prostatectomy. Like radical prostatectomy, patients experience dry orgasms for life after treatment with IMRT and 3DCRT. The patient is given a PSA test several months following radiation to assess the effects of the radiation and the possible extent of his cancer. If the PSA level elevates over subsequent years following radiation treatment, then hormone therapy is usually the next best treatment option; a rise in PSA following treatment indicates recurrent disease. Approximately 25 percent of patients treated either by radical prostatectomy or radiation therapy will develop PSA recurrence within 3 to 5 years following initial treatment. It is possible for a few men to undergo salvage radical prostatectomy after radiotherapy as another option although some urologists are unwilling to perform that delicate surgery after external beam radiation therapy has been performed.

Brachytherapy

In the United States there are an increasing number of men with early stage prostate cancer receiving seed implantation instead of for surgery. This procedure for prostate cancer is being marketed aggressively in many clinics in the U.S. Radioactive seed implantation, or brachytherapy, is a treatment option extensively carried out in the United States, Canada, and in over 600 centres around the world for treating early stage prostate cancer; it is an alternative treatment to avoid either surgery or external beam radiation. Men are becoming more aware of the many complications and recovery time that follow surgery. Brachytherapy is not without its complications. Many urologists suggest that surgery for organ-confined cancer provides the best curative treatment and refer to radical prostatectomy as the "golden standard" because all the cancer is eliminated if the disease is organ-confined. However, radiation oncologists also believe that brachytherapy or improved external beam radiation technology provides equivalent curative treatment for patients with confined prostate cancer. Brachytherapy (brachy means "short" in Greek) uses radioactive seeds or pellets implanted into the prostate and delivers the radiation dose from a short distance within the prostate. Alexander Graham Bell, in 1903, first suggested the use of seed implantation for prostate cancer. Louis Pasteur, in 1911, suggested inserting the radioactive element radium in the prostate to eradicate the disease. The radiation oncologist uses the information from ultrasound study to develop special templates that will be used for implantation of seeds. Patients undergo CT scans and cystoscopy to determine the anatomy of the region and size of the prostate before seeding. Patients are prepared in advance of the procedure by consultations with a radiation oncologist.

The brachytherapy procedure usually starts with assessing the patient's prostate by performing ultrasonography. A computer stores the data and determines how many seeds are needed and where to place them. The first transrectal ultrasound-guided, template-guided implant procedure with iodine seeds was performed at the Seattle Prostate Institute in 1985 by Drs. Blasko and Ragde. These pellets or seeds are about 2.5 mm long and contain radioactive palladium or iodine. The radioactive elements iodine^{125} or palladium^{103} used for implantation are guided by ultrasound while the patient is under local or general anesthetic. Some radiation oncologists prefer to use the iodine 125 seeds because the spacing of those seeds is less critical than with palladium and the half-life of iodine is 60 days compared with 17 days for palladium. Palladium pellets give off energy faster than the iodine isotope. Half-life refers to the time it takes for half of the radiation to disappear. It takes about five half lives for the seeds to release most of the radiation. Palladium seeds are radioactive for about 85 days whereas iodine seeds are radioactive for about 300 days.

Pellets of the radioactive substance are injected directly into the prostate gland from a grid-like template placed between the scrotum and anus, or in the perineum area. The exact position for delivery of radioactive seeds into the prostate is determined ahead of time and a three-dimensional map of the prostate is made. The seeds also contain the precise amount of radiation for the patient. The seeding implant requires 24 to 32 needles with each needle carrying 3 to 6 seeds. The radiation dose depends on which radioactive seed is used – a higher dose of radiation is administered with iodine than with palladium seeds. The grid-like template guides the needles that will shoot between 50 and 150 seeds, depending on the size of the prostate and from findings of earlier tests on the patient. The peripheral zone of the prostate receives the highest concentration of seeds. You will recall that the peripheral zone is home to most prostate cancer cells or tumours. The implant is completed in about 45 to 90 minutes as an outpatient procedure under spinal or light general anesthesia. The patient is free to go home the same day or the day following brachytherapy. Some side effects include urinary frequency and urgency, rectal irritation, and erectile dysfunction rates are reported to be between 25 and 50 percent following seed implantation. It may take well over one year for a man to regain his sexual potency. Urinary tract irritation and urgency to urinate affect a high percentage of men after brachytherapy and the condition may persist for up to two years although most patients' symptoms are resolved within one year.

Who qualifies for brachytherapy or what is the patient's eligibility for brachytherapy? As with radical prostatectomy, men with organ-confined prostate cancer are eligible for brachytherapy treatment. A Gleason score of 7 or less and a PSA of less than 10, two positive biopsy cores, and T1c –T2c staging are acceptable criteria for brachytherapy as general guidelines. However, patient eligibility or criteria for brachytherapy may vary from one clinic to the next. Patients may be classified into low, intermediate and high risk for brachytherapy. Patient and risk factors may be considered for brachytherapy combined with hormone therapy or radiation therapy. The radiation oncologist makes the final decision on a man's profile based on his Gleason score and grade, PSA level, the volume of tumour as determined in the ultrasound, the number of positive biopsies, and the stage of the cancer. Brachytherapy patients take alpha blocking drugs to alleviate urinary retention starting before, during and after treatment. Men who have been treated for BPH with TURP may not be eligible for brachytherapy; TURP patients are treated with seeds placed mainly in the periphery of the gland. Patients with small TURP defects are eligible for implantation but the risk of incontinence may be high. Men with prostates smaller than 50 grams or 50 cubic centimetres may qualify for the procedure. Occasionally, a patient with a large prostate gland may be placed on hormone therapy to downsize the prostate volume before proceeding with treatment. There are some men who have very large prostate glands (over 60 cc in volume) who may not be good candidates as some complications may develop during the seeding process. It has been suggested that men who have a life expectancy of more than 20 years with organ-confined cancer should be discouraged from having brachytherapy because the long-term information on survival rates for brachytherapy is currently about 15 years. However, with the success of brachytherapy today, it seems unlikely that the outcome will worsen in the next five years. Men, 75 years of age or younger with organ-confined prostate cancer could qualify for brachytherapy.

After the brachytherapy procedure is completed many men are fitted with a urinary catheter; the recovery from the procedure is usually quick. The perineal region is iced to reduce any swelling and pain shortly after seeding. You may be discharged on the same day but you will be discouraged from driving a vehicle. Your doctor will tell you what you should drink, eat or avoid and the medication to take after being discharged. Since you are a radioactive, you should not be in close contact with pregnant women or have your grandchild sit on your lap for the next few weeks. Don't worry, the seeds eventually lose their radiation activity externally but remain active within the prostate. Palladium seeds are radioactive for 85 days and iodine is active for about 300 days. The physical seed encasing will remain permanently within the gland and is made of titanium but it is not harmful; titanium is often used for joint replacements. There may be a tinge of blood passing into the urine after the implant. Seek medical attention immediately if you have any profuse bleeding or blood clots.

Erectile dysfunction (ED) is commonly experienced following implantation and in most cases the incidence is lower than following surgery or external beam radiation. A five-year study on erectile dysfunction was conducted at Memorial Sloan-Kettering after brachytherapy and the reported incidence for ED was just over 50 percent. Another significant study conducted by Dr. Mabjeesh and colleagues in the International Journal of Impotence Research investigated sexual function after iodine seed implantation. Reports from the literature show that 6-53 percent of patients experience ED following brachytherapy. In men who were sexually active prior to treatment, potency rates after brachytherapy alone were high. Up to 80 percent of patients after 3 years were able to have adequate erections for satisfactory sexual intercourse with or without the modern drugs for treating ED. Dr. Merrick and others investigated brachytherapy-induced erectile dysfunction through a validated questionnaire on 226 men; they found that ED occurred in 50 percent of all patients at 3 years. For men less than 60 years potency was preserved in 61 percent; for men between 60 and 69 years potency was 49 percent and men older than 70 years, potency was 32 percent in the above study. A man's ejaculate will diminish and few men experience dry ejaculates after brachytherapy. As mentioned, urinary frequency and urgency are common but you have to be patient as it may take several weeks to restore normal urine flow; the rate of incontinence is low following brachytherapy. Some rectal bleeding and diarrhea may be experienced after seeding; constipation is also experienced and stool softeners are recommended. Flatulence is common so avoid eating beans that may add to the problem. On rare occasions, a seed may dislodge into the urine and it is recommended that after implantation a condom should be used to prevent any seeds from entering the vagina during sexual intercourse. The radiation oncologist will advise the patient on post-operative procedures, of any symptoms that may occur, and general precautions before the patient is discharged. The patient will be given a card to carry so as to inform anyone that he has been treated with a radioactive substance, especially when passing through security check points.

Drs. Haakon Ragde and John Blasko at the Pacific Northwest Cancer Foundation in Seattle reported a 10-year follow-up study, of the results of two groups of patients after brachytherapy: those who received seeding only were in the low risk group and the high-risk group received seeding plus supplemental external beam radiation. The low risk group (having low scores of PSA, Gleason grade, and tumour stage) who were treated with seeding only and who remained free from tumour recurrence had decreased by 19 percent. At 10 years of follow-up, 60 percent of all men were tumour free. Surprisingly, the tumour recurrence rate was higher in the low-risk patients who received seeding only than in the high-risk patients who received both seeding and external beam radiation. The latter study suggests that in the long term, seed implantation alone may not be a sufficient treatment for many patients with early prostate cancer. Another study conducted by Dr. Deger and colleagues in Germany administered high dose brachytherapy using iridium192 and 3D conformal radiation therapy for localized prostate cancer. The survival rates increased with low risk groups and the low risk group was defined as having initial PSA values of less than 10 ng/ml and T1c to T2 staging. Intermediate and high risk groups experienced significantly lower five-year survival rates than the low risk group. It appears that some patients undergoing brachytherapy should have a follow up session with external beam radiation for long term survival.

Hormonal Therapy

The basic role of hormones and the influence on the prostate was presented in Chapter One and summarized in Figure 1.3. It is important to know how the prostate gland responds to anti-testosterone therapy or androgen deprivation therapy and hormonal interactions. Testosterone is the male sex hormone produced by interstitial or Leydig cells in the testes; its production is under the influence of the hypothalamus and pituitary glands, located in the mid-ventral region of the brain. Testosterone is produced from puberty and throughout the life of the adult male but its level gradually declines as men age, even starting at an age of about 40 years. A significant number of men even without being treatment for prostate cancer or are asymptomatic may experience a loss in sexual potency at an age of about 50 years, and by 80 years of age about 50 percent of men become sexually dysfunctional. Testosterone is responsible for establishing the male secondary sex characteristics which include development of facial and body hair, the sex drive, deeper voice, receding hairline and baldness, increased muscular and bone development. Testosterone is converted into dihydrotestosterone (DHT) by using the enzyme 5-alpha-reductase in the prostate. DHT activates receptors in the nucleus of prostate cells to promote certain growth factors. Blocking testosterone production either by bilateral orchiectomy (castration) or with androgen deprivation therapy slows down prostate cancer cell activity, benign growth and reduces the progression of metastasis of cancer. Luteinizing hormone (LH) secreted from the pituitary gland, and gonadotropic releasing hormone (GnRH) such as luteinizing hormone-releasing hormone (LHRH) secreted from the hypothalamus, normally control the production of testosterone. Any drug used for androgen deprivation is meant to ultimately block or suppress testosterone directly or indirectly.

Estrogen preparations such as diethylstilbesterol (DES) may be administered to block testosterone levels as one form of hormone therapy. DES inhibits both LH and GnRH production and will suppresses testosterone production. It is important to ask your physician and pharmacist about the side effects of DES or with any other hormonal medication. DES may lead to fluid retention, swelling in the legs and could cause blood clots which may travel and lodge in your lungs, heart or brain. I should not have been prescribed DES as other androgen deprivation hormones were available and safer to use than DES. I developed a blood clot in my lungs while taking a one milligram daily dose before my surgery as neo-adjuvant therapy. After two days of intense pain on the lower right side of my chest, I decided to go to my primary care physician who recommended an X-ray. The X-ray came in negative but the pain continued and I occasionally coughed up tiny amounts of blood. My physician called my urologist who recommended that I have a lung scan done immediately and the results showed a blood clot or thrombosis in my right lung. That was a very scary experience and it was indeed a close call for me. The next day I was admitted to have anti-coagulant treatment as blood clots can be fatal! I recall that DES was used in the early 1960s with steers to make them grow bigger and increase their carcass weight for market. DES was since banned by Agriculture Canada. I was put on warfarin (an anticoagulant) for an extended period of time to remove any blood clots and had to take some time off work. Dr. Chaudhary and colleagues reported that men taking 3 mg/day of DES in a randomized trial involving patients with metastatic prostate cancer, 33 percent developed cardiovascular or thromboembolic complications. Low levels of DES are administered in conjunction with other anti-androgens in some jurisdictions but I discourage anyone from taking DES as serious vascular problems can develop. The reason for taking DES before surgery, as far as I understand, was to down size the tumour and prostate and suppress testosterone levels. It did not downgrade the tumour but it did downsize my prostate. As far as I can tell, DES is no longer recommended by urologists and oncologists in Canada and should never be prescribed.

Flutamide, bicalutamide and **nilutamide** are anti-androgen drugs that work by preventing the male hormones from attaching to the androgen receptors in prostate cancer cells and from stimulating their growth. There are side effects too with using flutamide, bicalutamide or nilutamide, and these include decreased sex drive, gynecomastia or breast enlargement, nausea and possible liver damage. Flutamide (Eulexin), bicalutamide (Casodex) and nilutamide (Anandron) are used in combination with agonists like luteinizing hormone releasing hormone or LHRH. Another effective anti-androgen is **cyproterone** acetate or Androcur (steroidal) and may be administered to patients with prostate cancer. Cyproterone also targets the hypothalamus to inhibit LHRH production and lowers LH production, thus reducing testosterone levels.

In my opinion, the best approach I am aware of to achieve safe and effective androgen blockage is by using **LHRH agonists** which are similar, but not identical to, LHRH that the hypothalamus normally produces. LHRH agonists include Zoladex (goserelin) and Eligard (leuprolide) that initially cause a temporary testosterone surge for about ten days (the "flare effect") by stimulating the pituitary gland. An LHRH agonist after the temporary surge is over inhibits LH and disrupts the pituitary-testicular pathway, shutting down testosterone to castrate levels. Doctors often prescribe flutamide or bicalutamide to block the initial testosterone surge;

that initial surge increases testosterone levels that will produce the negative effect of what the anti-androgen therapy is supposed to achieve. Bicalutamide, an anti-androgen drug, is also administered along with LHRH analog and is used to control advanced prostate cancer. Of course, having an orchiectomy as a viable option for an older man is a very safe way to remove most of the circulating testosterone. One study reported by urologist Gleave and colleagues of patients having neoadjuvant hormonal therapy using leuprolide and flutamide before having radical prostatectomy found that "ongoing biochemical and pathological regression of tumour occurs between 3 and 8 months of neoadjuvant therapy…." A significant drop in PSA value was realized as well as a decrease in prostate volume. Dr. Gleave and colleagues also reported that eight months of neoadjuvant androgen withdrawal therapy "results in low positive margin rates and PSA nadir levels" as well as decreasing tumour volume. It should not be concluded that 3 months of neoadjuvant therapy is superior to 8 months or vice-versa.

LHRH agonists are available as subcutaneous injections below the skin in the abdominal area or buttock muscle every 2-6 months and may be administered only once before surgery. Administration of these agonists is also given to patients with advanced cancer. Be aware that these drugs are very expensive but cancer patients in Canada receive these drugs free of charge. Some urologists, but not all, recommend administering LHRH agonists prior to the patient having surgery. The main role of anti-androgen treatment is *combined androgen blockade* of testosterone from the testes, androgens from the adrenals, and dihydrotestosterone from its receptor sites in the prostate. LHRH agonists seem to do their work by binding to receptors between the hypothalamus and pituitary glands. LHRH agonists work in the same way as orchiectomy, a form of medical castration. Be warned that after prolonged hormonal treatment, prostate cancer may not respond to anti-androgen therapy and hormones may become increasingly ineffective. Cancer can, therefore, become resistant or non-responsive to continued hormonal treatment. Hormonal treatment on its own is not curative for prostate cancer.

A so-called innovative approach to hormonal treatment is by intermittent means, and is advocated by some oncologists and urologists. Drs. Pether and Goldenberg at the Prostate Centre in Vancouver reported that *intermittent androgen suppression* affords "an improved quality of life when the patient if off therapy, with reduced toxicity and costs…intermittent therapy will become an alternative to radical prostatectomy or irradiation for primary treatment of localized prostate in older men with a life expectancy of less than 10 years." Dr. Sharifi and colleagues in an article in *JAMA* reported that there is no proof that intermittent androgen deprivation therapy would prolong the survival of the patient compared to continuous treatment. The final outcome of combined androgen blockade whether it is intermittent or not is still not very clear. Urologist Walsh stated that "no form of hormonal therapy delays progression of disease. The only thing it delays is your knowledge of this progression." But Dr. Walsh added that hormonal therapy eases many symptoms of advanced prostate cancer cases. Urologist Scardino also cautioned that "intermittent therapy offers a false promise that men can enjoy more time free of the side effects of hormone therapy." One of the pioneers of intermittent hormone therapy, Dr. Nick Bruchovsky, spoke about the long-term tumour control of prostate cancer and a decline in mortality rate. Continuous androgen deprivation leads to non-responsive of cancer tumours, thus intermittent androgen deprivation may provide some benefits to advanced cancer patients. The quality of life is improved when the patient is on the "off" period rather than on continuous hormone treatment.

Orchiectomy or surgical removal of the testicles remains one last option in order to remove all testicular testosterone which feeds the prostate gland and tumours. There would be no need to have hormonal therapy if a man is surgically castrated and without experiencing the side effects of taking anti-androgens. There are some significant side effects after an orchiectomy and these include loss of sex drive, breast tenderness and enlargement, loss of bone density and hot flashes. Less than 5 percent of adrenal androgens such as androstenedione affect the prostate gland thus removal of testosterone by surgical castration is the major hormone to be concerned about in advancing prostate cancer. Cyproterone acetate has been used in conjunction with castration in some clinics for total androgen blockade. In an article in *Our Voice* (a publication on prostate cancer in Canada), one patient who had brachytherapy had his PSA escalate to 18 ug/l. He was then put on cyproterone but had terrible reactions to the drug. His urologist suggested removal of his testicles. The patient wanted another opinion and wrote to Our Voice for advice on whether castration should be done. The response was in the affirmative, and the magazine suggested castration or an orchiectomy. If you have an orchiectomy, be sure that you ask about side effects and possible medications to take in the weeks and months that follow. Hormonal therapy or testosterone deprivation does not provide a cure for prostate cancer, but it does down-size the prostate volume and perhaps down-stage the tumour before radiation or following aggressive treatment. For advanced prostate disease, combined androgen blockade therapy is eventually going to stop working because hormones will have little effect on the cancer. Dr. Patrick Walsh commented that "there has been no convincing scientific evidence to prove that early hormonal therapy prolongs life. Hormonal therapy does not cure prostate cancer."

Always ask questions about the effects of prescription drugs when you pick up your medication. It is also a good idea to remain with the same pharmacy as the pharmacist can easily access your medication on computer. You should also remind your pharmacist of any other medication you are currently taking since any new drug being prescribed may interact with other medications or may be harmful in combination. Doctors may not know as much as the pharmacist about the use and side effects of certain drugs, so it is important to get as much information from your pharmacist as well as from your physician. Finally, keep in contact with your regional Cancer Centre or Agency and find ways to reduce the cost of drugs or to receive them for free if you are not on an extended medical plan or you cannot afford to purchase them yourself. Oncologists at Cancer Clinics in Canada will advise patients about drugs that are covered by the provincial health care systems.

Alternative Treatment Approaches

Chemotherapy has been found to be generally ineffective in treating prostate cancer. However, many good responses can be achieved with chemotherapy and with selected experimental drugs currently being tested. Many drugs have been tested in laboratories and used to treat different cancers. The drug docetaxel was discussed earlier as being effective in reducing cancer from spreading outside the prostate capsule. Dr. Chaudhary and colleagues in the U.S. reported that docetaxel, in combination with prednisone, and docetaxel in combination with estramustine, have been shown to improve survival in patients with metastatic androgen independent prostate cancer. Dr. Tannock found that when docetaxel was given once every three weeks with prednisone there was superior survival and improved rates of response in terms of pain and quality of life in advanced prostate cancer patients. Chemotherapeutic agents continue to be used for advanced prostate cancer and some men have derived benefits from this form of treatment. A prostate cancer trial in Canada using docetaxel as a chemotherapy agent for breast cancer found that it reduced the size of the prostate cancer and can reduce the risk of having cancer at the prostate margins. Calcitriol, a form of Vitamin D, has recently shown promising results when combined with docetaxel. A large clinical trial with calcitriol and docetaxel is now underway in an American Cancer Society study. *Radioactive strontium*[89] radionuclide, consisting of beta particles is administered intravenously to relieve pain in the bones for advanced prostate cancer and is known to curtail the growth of bone metastases. Combination therapies such as strontium[89] and docetaxel are presently being explored in clinical trials to treat bone metastases with pain in advanced prostate cancer. Other chemotherapeutic drugs such as doxorubicin with strontium89 showed longer survival in patients compared to those who took doxorubicin alone. The combination of neoadjuvant docetaxel and neoadjuvant hormone therapy in conjunction with radiotherapy on high risk prostate cancer patients provided successful results according to oncologist McKenzie.

Many new drugs are being developed to help patients deal with pain when the cancer has metastasized and progressed away from the pelvic region. External beam radiation is also widely used to treat bone pain. Biphosphonates are a powerful class of drugs administered by injection to inhibit bone deterioration, reduce bone pain, and may also be used to prevent bone fractures. The new drug zoledronic acid, a biphosphonate, was approved in Canada to treat prostate cancer patients. A significant number of men receiving androgen-deprivation therapy for advanced prostate cancer developed bone fractures in a comparison study done by Dr. Shahinian and others. Drugs that reduce bone fractures will be useful for patients on androgen deprivation treatment. A chemotherapeutic agent called mitoxanthrone together with cortisone pills alleviate pain in advanced prostate cancer patients. It is well known that when advanced prostate cancer has metastasized in the bone the patient experiences excruciating pain. The purpose of treating patients with advanced prostate cancer is to maintain a good quality of life, reduce progression of disease, relieve symptoms and prolong life.

Endothelin is a vasoconstrictor (narrowing of blood vessels) substance and is linked to bone damage when bone becomes thick and hard with cancerous cells. Endothelin blocking agents have shown promise in alleviating pain in advanced cancers of the bone. An experimental vaccine developed by scientists at Johns Hopkins Medical School is being tested on a few patients with prostate cancer; the results from this vaccine trial are unavailable at this time. One experimental vaccine removes cells from the immune system and exposes them to prostate specific membrane antigen (a "foreign protein"). These cells are put back into the body where they induce other immune cells to attack the prostate cancer. Several approaches used in cancer vaccine development are designed to stimulate the body's own immune system to fight cancer. An experimental vaccine was tried on 19 men in Britain and reported in the *British Journal of Cancer.* Researchers reported that the experimental vaccine slowed the rate of PSA increase. One controlled study in Britain tested the effectiveness of a vaccine against the human papilloma virus that causes cervical cancer. It included 12 167 women aged 16 to 23 in 13 countries. The vaccine Gardasil was effective against advanced-stage abnormalities of the cervix that lead to invasive cervical cancer. To my knowledge, no controlled studies have been done in vaccine trials for prostate cancer but you may expect to learn more about vaccines in preventing the incidence of certain cancers. Monoclonal antibodies are being used to attack prostate cancer cells; to date there are no data available for using antibodies to treat prostate cancer. Radioactive isotopes can be made to tag onto monoclonal antibodies and directed to specific targets in the body; this method was used effectively to shrink lymphomas.

Microwave thermotherapy is still experimental for treating prostate cancer using guided ultrasound. Both the rectum and urethra remained at a safe temperature but the prostate is heated to a cytotoxic temperature of 55° Celsius. Dr. Sherar and others concluded that the treatment is safe even with recurrent disease after external beam radiation. Dr. Sherar cautions that further studies are needed but microwave thermotherapy is an option for recurrent disease and for treating primary prostate cancer. New drugs are now being used as *angiogenesis inhibitors* by attacking the new blood vessels being formed by malignant cells. Keeping any new blood vessels from developing is another way to stop the spread and growth of cancer cells. Many new blood vessels are formed and needed to nourish cancer cells; cancer cells that are deprived by severing the blood supply eventually die. A protein known as *thrombospondin* was discovered that inhibits blood vessel growth and regulated by p53 oncogene; it is speculated that mutations in p53 may turn off that protein resulting in angiogenesis and further promote tumour growth. The role of *statins* to reduce blood cholesterol levels is also known to reduce tumour growth including prostate cancer. "There is increasing evidence that statins are synergistic with other chemopreventive agents...that lovastatin induced a five-fold increase in apoptosis in colon cancer cells" as reported in *Oncology* journal by Dr. Stamm. A report from Children's Hospital in Boston stated that "epidemiologic studies have begun reporting that people taking cholesterol-lowering drugs have a significantly reduced incidence of prostate cancer and other cancers." A report from the Urological Research Foundation identified a protein found on the cell membrane known as hepsin; this protein may activate a growth factor that causes prostate cancer cells to multiply. Research was done with mice without *hepsin* and they developed normally. If an inhibitor of hepsin was developed it may have promise in controlling prostate cancer and as a means of chemoprevention therapy. This information on treatment options is not in any way recommended as medical advice for patients. Talk to your doctor about the best treatment options for you.

Objectified Active Surveillance

I mentioned earlier that a physician may decide to do nothing for a man who is 75 years of age or older and with accompanying health problems such as diabetes, cardiovascular disease or has suffered from a stroke, and with a well differentiated and confined malignant prostate tumour. The practice of watchful waiting, by monitoring his cancer or by *objectified active surveillance,* is an option for such as person with periodic testing, including a biopsy. If the cancer shows any signs of increased activity or progression after some time of active surveillance, the oncologist or urologist will recommend appropriate treatment. As mentioned earlier in one study, up to 40 percent of men over 70 years of age had localized prostate cancer when autopsies were conducted for other causes of death. *Most men will die with but not of their prostate cancer.* In a Swedish study conducted by Dr. Johansson and colleagues, 223 patients with early stage prostate cancer received *no treatment* or were on watchful waiting but patients with tumour progression were treated with hormones. The observation period was 20 years and the investigators found that most cancers had an indolent course during the first 10 to 15 years. A follow-up from 15 to 20 years showed a decrease in overall survival rate. This study supports radical treatment, especially for patients with a life expectancy exceeding 15 years.

Men whose life expectancy was less than 15 years may be better served with active surveillance. A Scandinavian study in a randomized trial of 695 men of a mean age of 65 years compared *radical prostatectomy with watchful waiting in early prostate cancer* for a duration of 10 years. *The first report* of that study found that "radical prostatectomy significantly reduced disease-specific mortality, but that there was no significant difference between surgery and watchful waiting in terms of overall survival." *Three years later,* a follow up study by Dr. Bill-Axelson and colleagues reported in the *New England Journal of Medicine* that "radical prostatectomy reduces disease-specific mortality, overall mortality, and the risks of metastasis and local progression. The absolute reduction in the risk of death after 10 years is small, but the reductions in the risks of metastasis and local tumor progression are substantial." Active surveillance has not been shown to prolong a man's life with early prostate cancer and earlier radical treatment is advisable especially for younger men, but it may allow older men to avoid the side effects of aggressive treatment without compromising their life expectancy.

Most prostate tumours grow very slowly. It takes many more years for cancer to become life threatening, developing from the cellular level to the tissue and then tumour level. Dr. Albertsen's study in *JAMA*, following conservative management by watchful waiting and androgen withdrawal therapy with 767 men aged 55 to 74 years in a U.S. study of men diagnosed with localized prostate cancer between 1971 and 1984 is of interest. The study found that men with a Gleason score of 2-4 had a minimal risk of dying from prostate cancer during 20 years of follow up. Men with a Gleason score of 5 or 6 tumours had an intermediate risk of dying from prostate cancer, and men with a Gleason of 8-10 had a high probability of dying from prostate cancer within 10 years of diagnosis. Men with low-grade tumours (Gleason 2-4) may be better served by conservative management or androgen withdrawal therapy rather than by aggressive means, even after 20 years of management. Dr. Albertsen and colleagues concluded that "the annual mortality rate from prostate cancer appears to remain stable after 15 years from diagnosis, which does not support aggressive treatment for localized low-grade prostate cancer." *Slow growing variants* of prostate cancer have PSA values under 10, PSA doubling times of greater than 4 years, and a PSA velocity of less than 0.75 ng/ml/year. The Gleason score in patients with the latter conditions often turns out to be 3+3, according to Dr. Strum. Adding other factors, such as tumour volume and clinical stage, may allow patients with those features to be considered as candidates for active surveillance.

Younger men or those in good health with localized prostate cancer under 70 years of age are suitable candidates for aggressive treatment and not by conservative means. Men with the conditions described above need to consult with an urologist and oncologist and to find out what treatment options are available – either active surveillance or aggressive treatment. Watchful waiting does not mean doing nothing, but actively monitoring the condition and any progression of prostate disease. He will then opt for an appropriate treatment when his condition shows any change and before his cancer becomes life-threatening. For men with indolent prostate cancers and a short life expectancy, watchful waiting or careful surveillance of their condition makes more sense than treatment by aggressive means. The decision to opt for active surveillance is based on knowledge of the patient's prostate and health profile. Dr. Whitmore asked the famous question, "Is cure possible in those in whom it is necessary, and is it necessary in those in whom it is possible?" How much longer would the average 70 year old man live with accompanying health problems? His average life could extend from 10 to 15 years, and by not having aggressive treatment with accompanying health related concerns he could enjoy a better quality of life by actively monitoring his prostate condition. Early detection of prostate cancer with PSA testing may offer a chance for a cure in men when it is possible and necessary.

If Prostate Cancer Returns

Radical prostatectomy and modern radiation therapy or brachytherapy are highly effective in treating prostate cancer yet "between 25 and 40 percent of patients will eventually have recurrence of the disease...," according to urologist Scardino. Most recurrent prostate cancer occurs within 5 years of treatment. With recurrent disease, when detected by a PSA rise after surgery, it is important to know if a man's cancer has gone into the lymph nodes or if it is in the seminal vesicles. One study at Johns Hopkins by urologist Partin found that a small percentage of men with elevated PSA following surgery had their cancer return locally in the prostate bed. However, with recurrent elevated PSA after surgery, a significant number of patients had distant metastases of their cancer. A doubling of PSA after one or two years following surgery and a Gleason score of 8 or more are important indicators of a high chance of nodal or distant metastases. The rate at which the PSA rises is an important indicator of disease progression after surgery or radiation. If the PSA doubles in less than 10 months, the disease progression is more serious. If the PSA doubling time is greater than 10 months, say two years, it may indicate local recurrence of cancer. This information is from Dr. Scardino's book, *Prostate Cancer.* Your doctor may want you to undergo further tests including a bone scan, a CT scan or an MRI. Promising results with the new ProstaScint scans to detect prostate cancer in the lymph nodes have been reported but not all oncologists believe the procedure is without concerns. A ProstaScint scan is like a bone scan and it involves injecting a low level of radioactive material to find prostate cancer that has spread beyond the prostate. The radioactive substance is attached to a monoclonal antibody (a type of synthesized protein) that sticks to prostate-specific membrane antigen, found in normal and cancerous cells. Lymph node cancer has been detected with some degree of success after the patient has been scanned by a gamma camera following a ProstaScint test. A new technique using the fusion of CT or MRI imaging with ProstaScint optimizes the images. The presence of lymph node and distant metastases cancers will allow for better treatment when the technique becomes more refined and widely available.

Doctors want to know the extent of a man's cancer before an optimum treatment is offered. Patients with a Gleason score of 8 or higher, positive lymph nodes, or positive seminal vesicles, or a PSA recurrence within the first year following surgery rarely benefit from radiation therapy, according to urologist Jeffery Cadeddu. External beam radiation and hormonal therapy are still appropriate even if the cancer has escaped the prostate bed. With elevated PSA scores after surgery, information about doubling time in the first year and the results of a Gleason score, it is possible to predict the probability of developing or not developing metastases within a given time. Urologist Pound and colleagues at Johns Hopkins in a study of 1997 men found that metastasis free survival was 82 percent 15 years following surgery. A detectable serum PSA of at least 0.2 ng/ml is evidence of biochemical recurrence. Oncologists and urologists generally reassure men with recurrent PSA to detectable levels that they should not panic. An analysis of a man's condition after surgery and his PSA doubling time or the time in months or years it takes for the PSA to return to detectable levels are guiding principles in deciding what follow up treatment the patient should undergo. Hormonal therapy or bilateral orchiectomy with chemotherapy are some of the options if distant metastasis of cancer is confirmed. A man will still have many years to live with distant metastasis if he undergoes appropriate treatment. Obesity is known to have a negative role in biochemical failure. Dr. Sara Strom and investigators studied 526 patients following radical prostatectomy and measured their body mass index (BMI) as a measure of obesity. In a 54-month follow-up, 18 percent of patients experienced biochemical failure but those with a BMI equal to or greater than 30 had higher rates of biochemical failures than non-obese men.

When patients have had radical prostatectomy procedures, it is possible to put them into four risk groups for recurrent disease as documented in Dr. Walsh's book, *Surviving Prostate Cancer.* First, men with a Gleason score of 6 or less and with or without capsular penetration but negative surgical margins have an *excellent chance* of undetectable PSA at ten years. *Second,* patients with a Gleason score of 6 and with positive surgical margins have a *good probability* of having undetectable PSA at ten years. *Third,* men with a Gleason score of 7 and with capsular penetration and positive margins, or a Gleason score of 8 and seminal vesicle invasion have a *moderate probability* of undetectable PSA at ten years. And *fourth,* patients with cancer in the lymph nodes have a *low probability* of undetectable PSA at ten years. These probabilities seem to make sense based on the progression of the disease. Detectable PSA levels appear to be an important factor for recurrent disease. With the advent of PSA testing, both the total and free PSA, most men who have had surgery fall into the first two scenarios above. With early detection of his cancer that is confined to his prostate, a cure by having surgery or brachytherapy is highly probable. Monitoring the PSA levels after surgery or radiation for several years is necessary to detect if any prostate cancer is likely to return. An undetectable PSA after 10 years is an excellent sign that a man has been cured of his cancer; however, doctors may advise patients to continue to have PSA tests for at least 12-15 years following surgery or radiation.

An ultrasensitive PSA assay addresses the early detection of recurrence of prostate cancer. It allows for a lower limit of detection of less than 0.01 ng/ml, resulting in earlier detection of biochemical relapse. Men with a nadir (lowest point) of greater than 0.04 ng/ml have an extremely high likelihood of relapse according to Dr. Shen in an article in *The Journal of Urology*. Ultrasensitive PSA nadir accurately predicts the risk of early biochemical relapse following radical prostatectomy. The third-generation ultrasensitive PSA assay detects earlier recurrence of disease following definitive treatment. After surgery or radiation, a man should have a PSA test after three to four months and subsequently every six to ten months. Higher risk patients (those with higher Gleason scores and grades) should be tested more frequently with the PSA. So what should you do if the PSA returns to detectable levels after one to five years following surgery or radiation? For recurrent disease with intermediate or lower risk patients, external beam radiation would be recommended after surgery when PSA levels start to rise to detectable levels. Some cancer cells may still be in the prostate bed but other cancer cells may have already gone astray and they are difficult to detect. When the entire history of the patient is known, it would be up to the oncologist or urologist to determine the next course of treatment. Options include radical prostatectomy (rarely done after external beam radiation), androgen deprivation, chemotherapy, radiation therapy. Should high intensity focused ultrasound, an alternative salvage therapy after external beam radiation or brachytherapy, be considered? If brachytherapy or external beam radiation were done, would cryotherapy be a beneficial salvage therapy. Those questions can only be answered by the patient and his physician.

For postoperative radiotherapy for recurrent treatment, favourable features would include a low PSA at the time of treatment, a slowly rising PSA, lower Gleason grade and a lower prostate tumour volume after pathology. Unfavourable features would include seminal vesicle invasion, lymph node metastases, a high or rapid rise in PSA, an initial tumour volume greater than 20 percent, and a high Gleason grade. A few patients that fall under the "unfavourable profile" may respond well to radiotherapy that may reduce the spread of prostate cancer. There appears to be a distinct benefit for adjuvant radiotherapy with long-term follow up. Dr. Catalona and colleagues reported that after surgery "adjuvant radiation therapy in patients with unfavorable pathology was significantly associated with better recurrence-free survival." Dr. Stephenson and others report-

ed similar findings of patients with high-grade disease or rapid PSA doubling time may achieve a "durable response to salvage radiotherapy."

Information presented on treatment options in this book is not intended to replace the advice of doctors and trained health professionals.
Furthermore, the opinions expressed represent my personal views and
from the research and studies cited in the literature.

Summary

More patients are being treated for prostate cancer with modern radiation therapies such as the three-dimensional, intensity modulated radiotherapy and brachytherapy. A high percentage of men experience recurrent disease after radical prostatectomy; salvage external beam radiation
therapy is known to provide a cure to many patients that experience recurrent disease especially those who have extra-capsular cancer including
seminal vesicle and lymph node metastases. Brachytherapy provides an
alternative to men who do not wish to have surgery and whose prostate
cancer is confined to the gland. Fewer complications are experienced after
brachytherapy as compared with surgery. Hormonal therapy continues to
be effective as neoadjuvant therapy before external beam radiation or radical prostatectomy. The prostate gland volume is down-sized and cancer
is suppressed with neoadjuvant and adjuvant hormonal therapy. For
advanced cancers, hormonal therapy has been shown to improve the quality of a man's life and prolong his life. Active surveillance of a man's
prostate condition remains an option for the patient with health problems,
with confined prostate cancer and a short life expectancy. Aggressive
treatment for such a patient's profile is not recommended as he will most
likely die with his cancer, not from it.

Chapter 10
Coping With Prostate Cancer

By reading this chapter you will learn:

- My experiences after being diagnosed with prostate cancer.
- Ways to cope with cancer and how to alleviate concerns and fears.
- About alternative and complementary care.
- Importance of Support Groups.

A Personal Journey

After my biopsy was performed, I was beginning to prepare myself for the worst and did not want to anticipate what the results from the biopsy might reveal. I wanted to block out the bad news. I decided to take a trip to the interior of British Columbia since it was my summer vacation, and in retrospect I realize I wanted to forget about the results from the biopsy. When I returned home there was a letter from my physician waiting for me. Why would my doctor write me a letter? My gut feeling was that something was wrong – doctors seldom write their patients, right? He wanted to see me as soon as possible and has written since his office had been unable to contact me by phone. I rushed to my doctor's office the next day. In the doctor's office we greeted each other as we had done on many previous visits. I have known him for many years and have always trusted his judgment and professional advice. I always felt that I was in good hands with my general practitioner. I happen to be his son's biology teacher, and we had previously talked about his son's excellent progress in my class. Our relationship was and continues to be good today. But the real issue at hand was the results from my biopsy and the urgency to see me; I felt my heart rate climbing above normal and experienced some suspense and anxiety while I sat in my physician's office. He opened my medical file after we were both seated and, after a brief pause which seemed like an eternity, came the dreaded words: "The biopsy showed that you have cancer." He did not procrastinate in telling me, as he knew that I always wanted a frank answer to any of my concerns; it was also the right way, and the professional way of breaking the news about my diagnosis. I sat there in disbelief, wishing that what I had heard was not true. I could not gather all my thoughts together at that moment nor could I think of anything to say or questions to ask as I was still in a state of disbelief, denial, and quite naturally confused and somewhat upset.

I was due to start my teaching two weeks later, in early September, and was beginning to be more concerned about my senior biology students rather than about the seriousness of my own cancer. I thought that I would have to leave my students mid-way through the semester and felt that by being away, I would disappoint them since they were in their final year and had to prepare for the provincial examinations. In retrospect, I'm not sure why I should have been so concerned about my students and my classes at the time of high anxiety and uncertainty about my condition. I should really have put everything else on hold until I got through my ordeal. I was "on pins and needles" and realized that I had to tell a few people about my condition and that I was still unaware of the course of my treatment. I did not know if my cancer was localized or if it had spread and no one had an answer to that question for me at that time. For a moment I thought that perhaps someone in the lab could have made a mistake with my tissues from the biopsy. Still wishing for better news, I kept asking "why me?" You get into a state of denial when confronted with the bad news of a cancer diagnosis. The next step was to get an assessment of my cancer from the urologist. One week later, I had that appointment to see him. My doctor told me that my urologist was very good and that he had completed his urology medical training at the Sloan-Kettering Cancer Center in New York. I was impressed with his medical background and was glad to know that he was a first-class surgeon who had done many operations for prostate cancer. I felt reassured that I was going to be in good hands.

Individuals respond in different ways to hearing of the shocking news that they have cancer. Men at a support group mentioned the following reactions to the news that they had prostate cancer: "End of the rope, radical change, what did I do wrong, fear, anger, death, side effects, quality of life, hope, anxiety." Those were a handful of comments from some men who were treated for prostate cancer in Vancouver. The psychological impact of learning this bad news can also be devastating, to say the least. You will need a great deal of support, perhaps even professional counselling, to ease the shock and pain of a cancer diagnosis. Your immediate family is one of the best support systems. You can also turn for support to close friends and colleagues you can trust at your workplace. There are some people whom you may postpone telling. For example, I waited to tell my 82 year-old mother, who was seven thousand kilometres away, until I visited her after my surgery and when I was in good health again.

Young children too may not deal well with learning the news of a mother, father or close relative being diagnosed with cancer, as they may not understand the implications, long or short-term, or the extent of the illness or even what cancer means. Caution and discretion should be used when informing younger children. My daughter was teaching English in Japan and returned to Vancouver after learning the news of my condition; she never returned to Japan but that was her decision, even though she knew that my surgery had gone well. My family and I had the occasion to take a vacation in the Caribbean before my surgery and the time with my family helped my frame of mind and was good therapy for me. Before we left on vacation I took my daughter with me to see my urologist, upon her request, and she asked him a few probing and pointed questions about my cancer and the impending surgery. I dare say that she seemed to be more concerned about my health than I was myself!

An important point to bear in mind is that good communication is needed when a family member is known to have been diagnosed with cancer. You have to be openly honest with your spouse or partner. Here are a few initial and basic skills for good communication: practice active listening and take time to know what your spouse is thinking or how she is feeling; take turns in the conversation, and avoid any blame or criticism. Tell your spouse how you are feeling, both emotionally and physically; the first time you break the news is not the last conversation you will have with your spouse or partner about your condition. However, do not allow your normal conversation to preoccupy yourself with your cancer – most of the time you should be talking about the normal daily things in your lives and plan ahead with normal activities in a positive way. With prostate cancer, for example, you should talk about your sexual relationship and what may be expected after treatment. Include your spouse in your treatment plans and take her to your physician so that both of you can share any information that is being provided. Continue to share any of your medical concerns before, during and after treatment with your spouse or partner; remaining silent when afflicted with an illness is not wise.

It is, of course, quite difficult to break the news of your diagnosis to young children. Children sense when something is wrong in the home and the need to break the news of mom or dad having an illness is important. Rehearse what you will say to your children and how to say it with your spouse. Keep in mind that cancer is a treatable disease. It is important to share any necessary medical information about your illness with your children and to use the word "cancer" in your discussion to avoid any misunderstanding. How do you explain the word cancer to a child? Perhaps start by showing drawings of cells that appear normal and those that have changed in cancerous cells. The Gleason grading scheme is a good way to explain how cells mutate from normal to abnormal types. When trying to explain how cancers develop, start by explaining how some cells change naturally and that no one knows why prostate cancer develops. Do not dwell on inheritance of cancer as that thought may not be well understood and may confuse children. You may start by mentioning that cigarette smoking brings about a change in the lungs, without getting into the details. You may also mention that diet, genetics and the environment play some role in promoting prostate cancer but that genetics is only a small part of the total equation. There is no need to show a lot of photographs depicting cancers; perhaps teenagers may respond more favourably to pictures of lung cancers with people who have smoked cigarettes as this strategy has been used as a deterrent with teenagers about the effects of cigarette smoking. You should not become too emotional when talking to a child about an illness. Children sometimes feel responsible for a parent's or sibling's illness. Explain, in as simple terms as possible, how cancer develops and do not scare them into thinking that it is contagious. Instead, mention that daddy or grandfather is getting the best medical help for his treatment. Be prepared for tough questions from your children or grandchildren and try and answer them honestly without giving any lengthy or detailed explanation. You may even have to say to your child that, "I will answer that question the next time I see my doctor as I do not have that information now."

Children, like adults, experience fear, anger, sadness and may naturally be confused when they hear about cancer. Tell them that it is normal for them to feel that way. Do not leave your child hanging on something that is puzzling or confusing, as it will create greater anxiety and worry. It may be important to consult with mental health professionals before you share the news with your children. Teenagers, unlike young children, need more information including a list of the tests taken, diagnosis and treatment. Entertain their questions and alleviate the fears that their lives will not change when mom or dad is being treated. Let them know that their normal routine will remain the same – going to the basketball games or school functions would continue. The American Cancer Society under "Additional Resources" at www.cancer.org recommends reading the book *Cancer in the Family: Helping Children with a Parent's Illness*. The National Cancer Institute (www.nci.nih.gov) in the U.S. has produced a booklet for teenagers titled *When Your Parent Has Cancer – A Guide for Teens*.

You are encouraged to join a prostate support group if you are diagnosed with prostate cancer and to ask your spouse or partner to attend the meetings with you. In fact, one prostate support group that meets in the evening is attended by spouses. All provinces in Canada and regions have organized *prostate support groups* where men are able to obtain information on a variety of cancer-related topics including nutrition, coping, treatment options and erectile dysfunction, to name a few. *The Canadian Prostate Cancer Network* has a website of useful information including an update on support groups and locations throughout Canada that can be accessed at www.cpcn.org. Both women and men in cancer support groups share personal experiences and important information. I have been associated with the Vancouver Prostate Support and Awareness Group (PSA) since 1994, a group specifically for patients with prostate cancer or for those who have been treated for the condition. Everyone is welcome to attend their meetings. The library at your Cancer Agency, public libraries, and Prostate Centres in an urban area may carry videos and up-to-date literature on prostate cancer. Support Groups generally invite spe-

212 Surviving Prostate Cancer

cialists to do presentations on relevant topics on prostate cancer, provide advice in promoting a healthier lifestyle, and other information. Refer to the list of useful websites at the end of this book. The Canadian Cancer Society also provides free informative booklets and pamphlets on the common cancers at www.cancer.ca. *Taking Time* is a booklet for people living with cancer and the people who care for them.

A prostate cancer diagnosis naturally comes as a big shock and has a tremendous impact on your psychological well-being. It takes time to accept the fact that you have a life-threatening disease; it is important to learn about available treatment options including palliative care for advanced disease. Many thoughts, some quite confusing, pass through your mind as you consider the best treatment options. In my experience, I wanted to learn as much possible about prostate cancer, about diagnostic tests and available treatment options. I found it a real challenge to get information on prostate cancer. I wanted to know more about a curative treatment plan. The information presented in this book will provide answers to some of your concerns. New therapies will emerge but the information presented in Chapters 7 & 9 on treatment options will remain reliable for some time in the future. Today, I am still interested in researching and learning more about this disease as there are still many unanswered questions. Knowing more about prostate cancer was one of the best therapies for me in order to cope with my condition as well as to explain my situation in an intelligent way to others. Mahatma Gandhi once said, "It is knowledge that ultimately gives salvation."

I have extensively researched several eminent medical and scientific journals and I used many articles in those journals for this book. I wanted to start by getting all the facts about prostate cancer because doctors do not and cannot provide you with all the information you need. Indeed, many doctors will not have all the answers to your questions. There is no quick fix to the list of problems and health concerns facing the individual after learning that one has been diagnosed with cancer. Some physicians may also give the impression that they do not have the time to discuss all your concerns. Be patient, as many of your questions will be answered eventually by your physician(s), by attending support groups or by doing your own research. I should add that patients in prostate support groups will not have the answers to your specific questions and their opinions may not be accurate or reliable.

I felt that acquiring information about prostate cancer made it easier for me to cope with my own situation, to make decisions about treatments and to understand some of the problems associated with having a radical prostatectomy. In Chapter 7, I listed a number of questions that you should be prepared to ask your urologist or oncologist as well as your general practitioner. After recovering from my surgery and feeling fit again following two months of surgery, I returned to my teaching and participated in activities sponsored by the Vancouver Prostate Support and Awareness Group. I also became a volunteer speaker for the Canadian Cancer Society for a short time.

How to Cope

In his book *Coping With Prostate Cancer*, Robert Phillips, a psychologist and director of the Centre for Coping, presents a detailed treatment and explanation of what a patient should know when diagnosed with

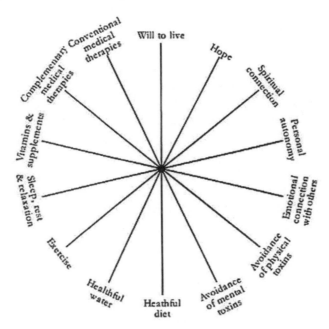

Figure 10.1: Healing and Recovery – spokes in a wheel model. With permission from the Centre for Integrated Healing, Vancouver, B.C.

prostate cancer or during the period of treatment. He suggests developing a positive mental attitude, laughing a little, deriving comfort from faith, making use of relaxation therapy, exploring professional counselling; the list of useful suggestions presented in his book for coping seems endless. The Centre for Integrated Healing (CIH) in Vancouver is staffed by medical doctors and other health care providers. The CIH bridges the gap between conventional and complementary cancer treatment. As part of their philosophy, the CIH recognizes that "illness" is not separate from "self" and supports the idea that "conventional medical treatment is just one spoke in the wheel of an integrated, holistic approach to healing." For more information about this cancer care model go to www.healing.bc.ca. The Newsletters posted on this website provide the summary research from medical journals and other useful information. The process of healing and recovery as shown in the "spokes in the healing wheel" below, include the mind and body. Take some time to study and if possible investigate alternate therapies; ask what should be avoided for a healthier lifestyle and select what is good for life's enjoyment.

Many people still believe that cancer is a death sentence but cancer is curable and preventable. About 80 percent of men diagnosed with prostate cancer survive. Some cancers can be cured or controlled for many years after diagnosis using a number of improved treatment methods as well as changing lifestyles. Keep in mind that most men die with, and not of, prostate cancer. If you smoke, stop, because cigarette smoke contains a multitude of carcinogens that will promote lung cancer and can eventually kill you as explained in Chapter 2. Lung cancer is still one of the biggest cancer killers and it is still the most preventable. Chapter 4 presented dietary consideration for preventing prostate cancer and for a healthier lifestyle. The Centre for Integrated Healing lists "10 Guidelines for a Healthier Diet" that reader may wish to access from their website.

Men are beginning to accept professional counselling as a form of therapy. It is a sign of strength and not one of weakness if you seek professional help when you are in a state of stress or depression. Women in general seem to be doing a better job in dealing with health related problems than most men. Cancer Agencies, the CCS, and other organizations such as the Centre for Integrated Healing have a staff to work with patients and conduct sessions on strategies such as relaxation therapy, music therapy, and other alternative therapies with cancer patients.

Meditation as an alternate form of therapy is also being encouraged by counsellors and health care professionals to reduce stress; exploring spiritual and religious beliefs have helped some people cope in times of stress and illness. People who have a faith perspective and strongly believe in prayer and engage in religious activities may derive some personal benefits by pursuing these practices. Prayer may be able to activate the immune system and increase the probability of recovery from illness; in my opinion, prayer does not offer a cure for your illness but for some people it reduces stress levels and offers contentment. The study of *psychoneuroimmunology* (how the central nervous system and our thoughts and emotions influence the physical health) needs to be explored further. Anyone who feels comfortable with prayer may derive personal benefits in his or her healing journey. Having spiritual values may allow some people to feel better; they may not be cured of their illness but prayer may alleviate symptoms of their illness. I do not want to sound callous, but it may well be that the placebo effect as documented in a few scientifically controlled studies may also work with prayer and having faith in the supernatural. The Centre for Integrated Healing provides the "self" model below that integrates lifestyle changes together with conventional treatment that contribute to the healing process; the road to recovery often requires more tools that conventional medicine can offer. You will recall the importance of intensive lifestyle changes in the prevention of diseases as discussed in Chapter 4. Some of those environmental factors are included below for active prevention of diseases including cardiovascular and cancer. Avoidance of toxins means freeing the body of the poisons in tobacco products and to avoiding drug and alcohol abuse.

You will find it necessary to make changes to your lifestyle before and after treatment. I continued to exercise moderately, golf and resumed occasional skiing in the winter. During the summer vacation, I plan to do more travelling, learn more about other cultures and visit wilderness areas on our fragile planet. I also believe that if you feel well you should continue working but it is also important to modify your work schedule if at all possible. A daily routine to follow is also good therapy – the axiom is to take one day at a time. You may not be able to attend all those meetings or do overtime work on the job and therefore you should not be afraid to say no to any unnecessary demands placed on your energy level as it will not be the same following treatment. It is important for people at your work to understand how you are feeling. You should not feel guilty for not performing at the same level as before – remember that you have just been through more than any other worker at your job site or office after having

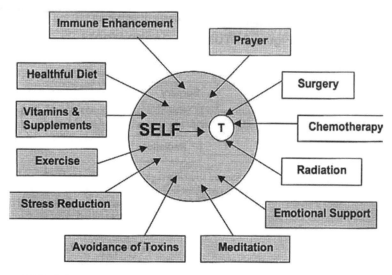

Figure 10.2: A Person-Based Model for Integrated Healing. With permission from the Centre for Integrated Healing, Vancouver, B.C.

major surgery or radiotherapy.

Your family is your greatest strength and asset. Friends, social events, a daily routine including work, your faith, daily moderate exercise, sensible nutrition with guided vitamin supplements and even a glass of red wine with dinner should be included for a healthy lifestyle. Many people are changing their eating habits by indulging in more vegetables and fruits and reducing their consumption of red meat and fatty foods. It is important to discuss with your physician the kinds of vitamin and mineral supplements that are needed. One well-known advanced prostate cancer survivor and philanthropist, Michael Milken, has funded *The Prostate Cancer Foundation* in the U.S. and has promoted a change of diet for preventing cancer. *The Taste for Living Cookbooks* by Chef Ginsberg and Milken provide recipes that Milken swears by for surviving his cancer. If you smoke, just quit for good! Life can be wonderful again!

The year following my surgery I decided to take early retirement from my high school teaching career. I am still keeping fit and belong to a gym.

After full-time teaching in a high school, I accepted a part-time position as a lecturer at a university to work with student teachers in their preparation to become classroom teachers. Retirement is not a good word to use for many who turn 65 years of age or older and who are still mentally and physically fit. By not working at a regular job or profession many new avenues or options are open for individuals to pursue even if you reside in smaller communities. It is necessary to keep mentally and physically active in order to maintain a good quality of life. Learn to pay attention to your body and dispense with thoughts that cause conflict. Life is too short to dwell on any negatives. Instead, focus on the ways you have always wanted to live, and live that life today!

Chapter 11
Guiding Principles

By reading this chapter you will learn:

- Guidelines for screening and detection of prostate cancer.
- Available support systems for patients.
- A brief guide to active living

The best advice is to have an annual physical examination including a digital rectal examination. You should have blood tests done for your general chemistry including diabetes, kidney and liver function. Other tests may be required depending on the condition of your health. Blood tests for cholesterol, low density lipoprotein (LDL), high density lipoprotein (HDL), triglycerides and hematology or components of whole blood are also recommended annual tests. Ask your doctor to order a serum PSA test for you even if you may have to pay for it yourself; if you want to know more about the PSA test review the information in Chapter 5 and in this chapter. Exercise of any form and a sensible nutritional plan should be part of your daily lifestyle. Also monitor your body mass index and waist circumference regularly.

What are the stated guidelines for having a PSA test? *The Canadian Urological Association* (CUA) states that the DRE and PSA measurements increase early detection of clinically significant prostate cancer; men should be made aware of the potential benefits and risks of early detection so they can make an informed decision as to whether to have this test performed. According to an Ipsos survey, 9 out of 10 urologists in Ontario always or often screen men by ordering a PSA test. Many more men seem to be requesting the PSA test, a wise decision if they are at risk or over 50 years of age. Another Ipsos-Reid survey carried out in British

Columbia, cited earlier, indicated that 50 percent of men aged 45 to 75 had a PSA test done in the past five years. *The American Cancer Society* and the *American Urological Association* recommend that both a PSA and DRE be offered to men beginning at 50 years of age and high risk men (with two or more affected first relatives for prostate cancer), including African-American men, may start testing at 45 years of age. In 2001, approximately 75 percent of men in the U.S. 50 years and older reported PSA screening and 54 percent reported regular PSA screening in a report cited by Dr. Thompson. Canadian men whose immediate relatives were diagnosed with prostate cancer and African/Caribbean Canadian men should also be screened at an earlier age. Several recommendations were suggested on PSA screening in the general population and discussed in Chapter 5. PSA screening has the advantage of identifying prostate cancer earlier while cancer is still localized and can be eradicated. The *Canadian Prostate Cancer Network* has "advised men in their forties to start a yearly regimen of PSA testing and digital rectal exams." On the other hand, the *Prostate Cancer Research Institute* in the U.S. strongly supports annual testing for the early detection of prostate cancer; it suggests that the PSA and DRE be done at age 35 for men with a family history of prostate cancer and for African-American men, and for all other men beginning at age 40.

The *Canadian Cancer Society* and the *National Cancer Institute of Canada* recommend that "all men should have the opportunity to undergo a PSA test if, after assessing the benefits and risks of PSA testing, they choose to have it. We therefore recommend that men should be made aware of the benefits and risks of early detection testing using PSA and digital rectal examinations." The Canadian Cancer Society (B.C. and Yukon Division) stated that the PSA test should be made available at no cost to men but borne by the provincial health insurance. The Canadian Cancer Society (CCS) funded a PSA screening study conducted in the Toronto area and reported in the August 2005 issue of *The Journal of Urology,* found that "screening of asymptomatic men with PSA was associated with a significantly reduced risk of metastatic prostate cancer." This finding seems to be very good news for men "because it suggests that early PSA screening may reduce the risk of metastatic prostate cancer" says Dr. Barbara Whylie of the CCS. Drs. Kopek and Goel authored this study and remarked that PSA screening may reduce the risk of death from this disease. This conclusion supports giving the PSA test to asymptomatic men and men who are at risk.

Prostate cancer today is discovered more often in young healthy males who can be treated successfully with modern therapies. Opponents of PSA screening believe that over-detection of small cancers in older men would cause unnecessary biopsies and their cancers would not prove to be a grave problem if left alone. An Ipsos survey in Ontario asked urologists if PSA screening results in significant over-treatment. The results were mixed: 48 percent agreed and another 40 percent disagreed. Active surveillance or monitoring of such a condition in an older man may prove to be beneficial when all tests results are known. The PSA test is not without inaccuracies in detecting prostate cancer; there are known false negatives and false positives in the general population. The free PSA is another diagnostic test that is highly recommended. It has some advantages over the total PSA test and should be done in conjunction with the total PSA as discussed in Chapter 5. The results from the free and total PSA tests would add meaning to diagnosis and prevent any unnecessary biopsy. A new screening tool has become available and is produced by Bostwick Laboratories in the U.S. It is called uPM3, a urine-based genetic test that is believed to be more accurate in detecting prostate cancer than the total or free PSA as confirmed by biopsy results. In the *Urology* journal of 2004, Dr. Fradet and others in their study concluded that "the overall accuracy of uPM3 was 81% compared with 40% for tPSA...and that uPM3 may provide some answers to current dilemmas of early prostate cancer detection..." The newer tests, such as the free PSA, the ultrasensitive third-generation PSA assay, and the uPM3 urine-based test may reduce the need for biopsies as those tests seem to perform better than the conventional total PSA alone in detecting the extent prostate cancer or its progression.

An appointment with an urologist or oncologist is advised if your primary care physician recognizes any abnormal changes in your prostate condition or if there is an elevated PSA reading or a suspicious PSA velocity rate or doubling time. The biopsy, under ultrasound guidance, is the definitive diagnostic procedure when clinical or laboratory findings indicate the possibility of prostate cancer. There is some disagreement as to the cutoff or threshold level of the PSA. You will recall in Chapter 5, Drs. Walsh, Catalona, Thompson and others recommended different cutpoints of total PSA values for a biopsy. Dr. Thompson and colleagues recommend that there should be no cutpoint for the total PSA but a continuum of prostate cancer risk exists for all values of PSA. You may want to consider the recommendations made about PSA cutoff values in Chapter 5, the use of the free PSA, and PSA velocity before having a biopsy.

As a general guiding principle, surgery appears to provide a longer survival advantage over other effective therapies; surgery is the preferred therapy for young healthy males with confined prostate cancer. Some younger men may wish to consider brachytherapy as an alternative to surgery. External beam radiation therapy provides excellent results for organ-confined cancer, extracapsular or cancer that has progressed within the pelvis or beyond as discussed earlier in Chapter 9. Men in their late 70s and 80s may be advised to have androgen deprivation therapy and active surveillance for cancer confined to the prostate gland. Of course, each situation is unique so you need to further consult with an oncologist and urologist. Men with comorbidities should avoid aggressive treatment. Weigh your decision based on the hands and experience of the specialist and the facility. It is also important to investigate whether your urologist has a good track record. What is the success rate of having brachytherapy versus radiation therapy or should both be performed? Is the cancer facility performing 3D conformal radiation therapy as well as intensity modulated radiation therapy? Is there a need to have adjuvant hormonal therapy and what is the advantage of neoadjuvant treatment? Should high intensity focused ultrasound or cryotherapy, two new treatment options now offered in Canada, be considered for your case? Have you, regardless of age, had all your questions answered before deciding on a specific treatment? You need to understand why a particular treatment option offers the best chance of a cure. What are the disadvantages and advantages of treatment X over Y? Although it may be difficult to predict any medical outcome with any accuracy, it is important to review the websites of the nomograms listed in this book for second opinions. As mentioned in Chapter 6, the *National Comprehensive Cancer Network* at www.nccn.org provides suggested treatment guidelines based on patient information and history. Finally, on positive and hopeful note, the *Canadian Prostate Health Council* emphasizes that "a diagnosis of prostate cancer is not a death sentence. Prostate cancer in its early stages can be cured. Even in advanced stages, treatment can greatly improve the quality of life and prolong life." For some patients, prostate cancer may be treated as a chronic disease by oncologists even when a cure is unlikely.

Your immediate family and close friends are good support systems when any serious illness occurs or before surgery or treatment. Continue with exercise programs before surgery or radiation and check with your physician for advice as to the kinds of exercises to avoid after your procedure and when to resume exercise. It is also very important to have the confidence and trust of your family physician, oncologist or urologist. You may want to obtain a second opinion with another urologist or to make an appointment to discuss your concerns with an oncologist. Also contact your Cancer Society or Agency in your province for advice to help answer any questions as well as for guidance during times of anxiety and need. Some prostate cancer patients benefit from joint counselling with their spouses or partners. I believe that knowing more about your disease through the research of the literature is an excellent form of therapy. I also found that the rapport with men at the Vancouver Prostate Support and Awareness (PSA) Group was encouraging to me following my surgery. In fact, you should attend the meetings of support groups before opting for any treatment and also following treatment. Men at the support groups openly discuss and share their concerns and personal experiences. However, medical advice should be provided by your doctors and trained health professionals. The Canadian Prostate Cancer Network is known as the voice of prostate cancer in Canada and their website at www.cpcn.org contains useful information on prostate cancer. I encourage you to access the information from this website and locate a nearby support group. Alternately, send your questions to the website above or to your nearest Canadian Cancer Society or Agency at www.cancer.ca. The Cancer Information Service of the CCS can be reached at 1-888-939-3333 and information is available in several languages. It is important to access only reputable websites for information on cancer including the ones listed in the back of this book.

With regards to nutrition, you should reduce the consumption of foods high in saturated fatty acids, eat more fibre foods including vegetables and fresh fruits with suitable vitamin supplements. I take a high potency one-a-day vitamin/mineral supplement including a low dose of aspirin and eat sensibly. There are many websites providing nutritional advice and some advocate increasing your alkaline food consumption for a healthier lifestyle. Your physician should be consulted as to what vitamin and mineral supplements to take, if any. Don't believe everything you read about dietary food supplements or of the usefulness of a particular plant derivative. Indeed, plants hold many of the key ingredients for treatment of many diseases including cancer– phytochemicals in plants provide many useful functions but some also have harmful properties. When we reach inside the medicine cabinet we are often reaching for a plant or its derivative. Of the 250 000 flowering plants, about 5 500 have been tested for pharmaceutical properties in the laboratory. Some people swear that by taking certain food supplements they will become healthier and feel better but they may also be experiencing the placebo effect. I am skeptical about consuming products sold in some health food stores because I know very little about their ingredients or chemical composition. Are you taking supplements? If so, are they medically tested in placebo-controlled experiments or are you relying on anecdotes or hearsay from a few individuals? Of course thousands of different plant species have been used as medicines by various peoples of the world, especially in developing countries. The first nation peoples have used countless plants for a variety of ailments and their work is being studied by ethnobotanists.

Quacks and frauds sometimes suggest what we should eat, drink or take as supplements. A **quack** can be defined as a pretender to medical skill or a person who talks pretentiously without sound knowledge of the subject. Some people, when faced with the prospect of chronic suffering or death, may be tempted to try anything that offers hope. Many educated people sometimes resort to worthless remedies. I urge you to visit www.quackwatch.org for more information. This site combats health-related frauds, myths, fads and fallacies. People selling products at health foods outlets or through the Internet generally do not have a pharmacological background and cannot advise on drug interactions. They may offer incorrect information in order to sell their products. There are thousands of products, including drugs that are sold on the Internet that should be investigated before purchasing. For example, you should know that taking aspirin, high supplements of Vitamin E and *Ginko biloba* at the same time are not recommended – these drugs can affect blood clotting mechanisms and especially before surgery. Consult your doctor and pharmacist about drug interactions and their effects. Stay with the same pharmacy so that your pharmacist will have your record of medication on the computer.

Data suggests that regular exercise can help reduce the risk of prostate and breast cancers. According to Dr. D.C. McKenzie, a medical doctor and exercise physiologist at the University of British Columbia, some studies show both positive and negative relationships of exercise and prostate cancer. He cited a Stanford study that demonstrated a reduction of 10 to 30 percent risk of reducing prostate cancer with regular exercises. Exercise affects the endocrine system by reducing testosterone levels and increasing the immune system that provides added protection against prostate cancer. Reducing body fat level with exercise and following a sensible diet also reduces the storage depot for potential carcinogens. The relative risk of mortality is directly related to factors such as low fitness levels, smoking, hypertension, high cholesterol levels and obesity. Exercise physiologist McKenzie claims that about 60 percent of Canadians suffer from "sedentary death syndrome" that leads to a host of diseases such as cardiovascular problems, diabetes, stroke, cancers and respiratory diseases. Exercise of any kind (walking, jogging, hiking, or swimming) and strengthening your muscles can help prevent cancers and other diseases. A large cohort study conducted by Dr. Giovannucci and colleagues at the Harvard School of Public Health concluded that men engaging in physical activity were less likely to be diagnosed with poorly differentiated prostate cancers of Gleason grade of greater than 7. They further stated that although the mechanisms on physical activity and the association with prostate cancer are unknown, their findings suggest that regular exercise could slow the progression of prostate cancer knowing the documented benefits and importance of exercise.

A National Geographic magazine article in November 2005, "The Secrets of Long Life", documents similarities of good habits among super seniors in widely separated regions that experience longevity. Seniors in Sardinia (Italy), Okinawa (Japan), and Seventh-day Adventists in Loma Linda, California among other practices, do not smoke, put their family first, keep socially active, eat fruits, vegetables and whole grains, and live longer and survive for over 100 years. These three regions are known to have high rates of centenarians and suffer fewer of the diseases that kill most people. Of course, good genetic heritage, a careful diet and daily exercise also help build a healthy lifestyle.

Alternative and complementary medical treatment options contribute to maintaining a good quality of life, including the process of self-healing, keeping mentally active, maintaining an awareness of your self and the "power of the mind." You may become ill at any chronological age and the process of aging should not be construed as a failure or weakness. The mind is not separate from the body and how we feel has an important effect on our healing process. As mentioned in the last chapter, the information presented at the website www.healing.bc.ca is helpful and provides a second opinion. The family unit and support groups help too. You can also conduct your own research, learn how to cope with both mind and body connection, learn to control your illness and you may even alleviate some of the fears that are associated with a cancer diagnosis. Someone once said *"People don't grow old. When they stop growing, they become old."* As a concluding thought from Dr. Deepak Chopra it should serve as a reminder for all of us that longevity is still an individual achievement; it comes primarily to those whose expectations are high enough to reach for it. And as a final exercise for you older men, find three photos of yourself, one when you were 5 years of age or younger, another in your twenties, and a current image. Examine and compare those three photos carefully placed side by side. How do you see yourself as you advance in chronological but not necessarily in physiological age? We notice the effects of aging on our physical appearance, and especially in our facial features or receding hairline or lack of hair, but we do not realize that the real life-altering changes reside in places we do not see. Finally, when you awake in the morning, plan on making the new day the greatest day of your life.

> Look to this day,
> For it is life,
> The very life of life.
> In its brief course lie all
> The realities and verities of existence,
> The bliss of growth,
> The splendor of action,
> The glory of power.
> For yesterday is but a dream
> And tomorrow is only a vision.
> But today, well lived,
> Makes every yesterday a dream of happiness
> And every tomorrow a vision of hope.
> Look well, therefore, to this day.
>
> (Sanskrit Proverb)

Glossary

Ablation: as in cryoablation is to get rid of something, by freezing the prostate gland; hormone ablation refers to get rid of the hormone testosterone that targets the prostate.

Accessory reproductive gland: tissues including ducts which play a secondary role in enhancing sperm activity - prostate and seminal vesicles.

Active surveillance: to monitor a man's condition with a DRE and/or PSA, and the need for a biopsy during conservative or no treatment for prostate cancer; once referred to as watchful waiting; delaying treatment until conditions or symptoms become more apparent.

Acute: having a disease of short duration, severe symptoms.

Adenocarcinoma: malignant tumour from a glandular structure such as the prostate; may be felt (palpated) as a hard tumour.

Adjuvant: therapy given after radiation or surgery; neo-adjuvant therapy such as hormone therapy is given before surgery.

Adrenals: a pair of glands located above the kidneys and produces a number of hormones including androgens; makes up 5 % of total body androgens.

Analog: a synthetic body chemical.

Anastomosis: as in the connection between bladder neck and urethral suture.

Androgens: male hormones necessary for male sex characteristics, male sex organ development and function.

Angiogenesis: when new blood vessels form that nourish cancer cells; some drugs block these news blood vessels from forming to starve cancer cells.

227

Antigen: a foreign substance, usually a protein that stimulates the immune system to react and produce antibodies.

Anti-androgens: a from of androgen deprivation to block testosterone.

Apoptosis: or programmed cell death when cells commit suicide.

Benign: not cancerous or malignant; it does not invade and destroy the gland or tissues.

Benign prostatic hyperplasia or BPH: non cancerous or non malignant tissues which invade the prostate gland, usually from the inside out. Hypertrophy refers to the increase in the size of the cells.

Biopsy: removal of a piece of living tissue (from the prostate) with a needle for microscopic or biochemical analysis; it is most important in diagnosing if cancer is present.

Bone scan: refers to a picture taken after gamma rays emitted from the bones; used to detect any cancerous area.

Bound PSA: PSA that is combined with proteins. Elevation of bound PSA may signal the presence of cancer.

Brachytherapy: a form of radioactive seed implantation inside the prostate

Cancer: an uncontrolled and abnormal growth or division of cells; refers to malignancy and can spread or metastasize in other parts of the body; prostate cancer may move into the lymph nodes and bones.

Capsule: for prostate cancer it is the outer prostate wall like the skin of a plum.

Carcinoma: see cancer and adenocarcinoma.

Castration: the removal of the testicles as one way to prevent testosterone action on the prostate; also known as orchiectomy or orchidectomy.

Catheter: usually a flexible rubber tube inserted into an opening, urethra or a wound, to drain fluids; inserted into the bladder base to drain urine after radical prostatectomy or TURP.

Cavernous: the nerve that is responsible for erectile function running on the right and left sides of the prostate to the penis.

Chemotherapy: using powerful drugs to treat advanced stage cancer or to reduce the cancer in its earlier stage.

Chronic: a disease of long-lasting duration; it does not refer to the degree of the severity of the disease.

CAT scan: a computerized X-rays of the body used to identify cross sectional abnormalities such as lymph node metastases.

Combined androgen blockade: hormone therapy that uses anti-androgen drugs with LHRH analog.

Comorbidities: usually in older men suffering vascular disorders, hypertension or diabetes that should be known before treatment.

Corpora cavernosa: the spongy mass of tissue in the penis that fill with blood during an erection.

Corpus spongiosum: a smaller mass of tissue surrounding the urethra in the penis and fills with blood during an erection.

Cryoablation: or therapy is by freezing the prostate until it becomes an ice ball and the thawing ruptures cancer cells.

Cyproterone: an anti- androgen used to suppress testosterone and may be administered to prostate cancer patients before surgery or radiation.

Cystoscopy: visual examination (with light conducting bundles) of the bladder and urinary tract with a cystoscope.

Diethylstilbesterol (DES): an anti-androgen used to suppress testosterone and may be administered to prostate cancer patients.

Digital rectal examination (DRE): method used by the inserting finger of the physician into the rectum to feel the prostate.

Dihydrotestosterone: an analogue of testosterone; formed in the prostate gland by the conversion of testosterone with the enzyme 5-alpha reductase.

Doubling time: the time required for the PSA to double.

Down-sizing: reducing the prostate volume by neo-adjuvant hormone therapy.

DNA: deoxyribonucleic acid consisting of genes in the nucleus of the cell and carried all the hereditary information.

Ejaculate: semen which consists of sperm and fluids mainly from the seminal vesicles and the prostate gland in a single ejaculation at the moment of sexual climax. Dry ejaculate means no semen is produced after excision of the prostate and seminal vesicles.

Ejaculatory ducts: the passageway for semen to be carried to the prostatic urethra during ejaculation.

Endocrine: refers to a gland which manufactures a hormone and secretes it into the blood for use elsewhere; LH produced by the pituitary targets the testes to produce testosterone.

Endothelin: a chemical believed to cause pain in advanced cancer. Drugs are used to block endothelin.

Epididymis: after sperm cells pass from the tubules of the testes, they mature in this twisted tube of about 5 -7 metres in length; it also acts as a storage site of sperm cells.

Erectile dysfunction: the inability to achieve and maintain an erection sufficient for vaginal penetration.

Estrogens: a group of female sex hormones known to establish female sex characteristics such as breasts and promote the development of sexual organs and regulate the menstrual cycle; it is antagonistic to testosterone, the male sex hormone.

Estrogen therapy: drugs that give temporary suppression of prostate cancer; some drugs may shrink the prostate and keep the cancer from spreading. Side effects are often common in men who are on estrogen therapy like DES.

Exocrine: a gland which secretes substances, not hormones, into a duct or tube like the prostate or salivary glands.

External beam radiation: high linear accelerators given 5 days out of 7 for about 6 – 7 weeks; cancer cells may be killed, side effects do develop.

False negative: a false report of a low PSA level when it should be elevated and cancer is present after further tests.

False positive: a false report (high reading) for cancer with the test such as the prostate specific antigen (PSA) when it should be a low reading.

Follicle stimulating hormone (FSH): is a hormone produced in both males and females in the anterior pituitary gland and targets follicular cells of the ovary to stimulate their growth; also stimulates the cells of the seminiferous tubule cells of the testis to promote sperm cell production.

Foley catheter: a catheter inserted into the penis and into the bladder anchored with a tiny inflated balloon to drain urine.

Flare: a brief rise in testosterone levels after LHRH analogs are given.

Flutamide: an anti-androgen non-steroidal drug used by cancer patients to suppress the effects of testosterone on the prostate - it targets the prostate.

Free PSA: the ratio of free to total PSA; it is not bound and if the percent is low then cancer is suspicious.

Gene therapy: inserting genes with viruses as carriers to target cancer cells.

Gleason score: a method of grading cancer cells from well (2-4) to poorly differentiated cancer cells (8-10) – Gleason ranges from 2 to 10.

Gonadotropic releasing hormone: such as LHRH (luteinizing hormone releasing hormone) secreted from the hypothalamus, regulates the secretion of luteinizing and follicle stimulating hormones in the pituitary.

Grade: refers to the progression of cancer cells from low to high or to poorly differentiated tissue as seen with a microscope; determines how abnormal cancer cells are.

Gynecomastia: the enlargement and tenderness of the breast, usually after hormonal therapy.

Hormones: may be proteins or steroids; in the case of males, testosterone is the steroid responsible for male sex characteristics, produced by the testes, an endocrine organ, and targets the prostate, skeleton and muscles; in females see estrogens.

Hyperplasia: an increase in the growth of cells in the prostate.

Hypothalamus: located in the mid-ventral side of the brain above the mid upper roof of the mouth; secretes releasing hormones and regulates the pituitary and sex organs; other functions include temperature control.

Impotence: erectile dysfunction or the inability of the male to maintain or initiate an erection.

Incontinence: your inability to control the voiding of urine; dribbles occur as loss of voluntary control of sphincter muscle.

Indolent: tiny tumours that pose no immediate risk

Interstitial cell: these cells are found outside the seminiferous tubules in the testes and produce testosterone; also known as Leydig cell.

Infarction: small localized dead tissue when blood supply is inadequate.

Infection: a condition created by pathogenic microorganisms and causing injury to tissues.

Intensity modulated radiation therapy (IMRT): a new form of external beam radiation and effective in targeting tumours with lower side effects.

Intermittent hormone therapy: men will take the hormone and then stop when PSA levels are low enough; therapy is repeated some months later and men are closely monitored for their cancer.

Isoflavones: phytochemicals in soy products that help to combat cancer.

Laparoscopic radical prostatectomy: uses a hand held procedure or robotic interface in the abdominal wall for surgically removing the prostate gland and other diseased features.

Libido: the intensity of the sexual drive.

LHRH agonists: a synthetic form of LHRH used to block LH and prevent testosterone production.

Lobes (of prostate): five bulbous regions that make up the prostate.

Luteinizing hormone: or LH, secreted by the pituitary gland targets the Leydig or interstitial cells of the testes to stimulate or regulate the production of testosterone.

Luteinizing hormone releasing hormone: or LHRH produced by the hypothalamus of the brain stimulates the release of LH and FSH.

Lycopene: an anti-oxidant found in red grapefruits, tomato paste, sauce, watermelons that fight oxidative damage.

Lymph node: small rounded bodies which fight infection, having white cells which stimulate the immune response of the antibody and cell mediated types; often a common site of cancer.

Malignant: a tumour that invades tissues and organs and progressively becomes worse if untreated; may result in death of patient.

Metastasis: the movement of cancer from one site to another, through tissues or blood.

Monoclonal antibodies: substances produced to tag, diagnose or treat prostate cancer.

Multifocal: cancer appearing in several sites in the prostate.

Neoadjuvant therapy: usually treatment before either surgery or radiation with hormone therapy.

Neurovascular bundles: containing nerves that run alongside the prostate necessary for erectile function; also contain blood vessels.

Nitric oxide: a substance that is released at nerve endings during an erection, causing the spongy tissues and muscles in the penis to relax.

Nomogram: mathematical model for predicting a disease stage or outcome.

Oncologist: a physician who is specialized in treating cancer; within this specialized area there are several sub-specializations, eg. radiation oncology.

Orchiectomy: the removal of the testicles or castration usually done to deprive the prostate of testosterone; sometimes referred to as orchidectomy.

Palliate: to relieve pain in advanced prostate cancer cases.

Palpable: a doctor's gloved finger feels a lump or nodule during a digital rectal examination or DRE.

Partin Tables: a nomogram to predict the course of disease from biochemical and pathology findings.

Perineum: the area between the anus and scrotum.

Peripheral zone: the major part of the prostate beneath the capsule where most cancers are detected.

Pituitary gland: located below the hypothalamus and controls many organs, glands and the body in general; secretes many hormones including gonadotropic hormones which target the ovaries and testes.

Phosphodiesterase inhibitor: such as sildenafil (in Viagra) that will facilitate an erection.

Placebo: the fake pill or one not containing the active ingredient but resembles the pill with the active ingredient, having a placebo effect.

Priapism: prolonged erections and can be harmful.

Prognosis: the prediction or conclusion of the course of a disease; likelihood of recovery from a disease.

Proscar (finasteride): as an anti-androgen used by some BPH patients to shrink the prostate and increase urinary flow.

Prostate gland: located at the base of the bladder and is a male accessory organ; produces substances necessary to nourish sperms and maintain male fertility. It accounts for over 40% of the ejaculate.

Prostate specific antigen: or PSA is a protein-carbohydrate complex made in the prostate gland; an elevated reading is an indication of prostate disorder, not necessarily the presence of cancer but could be a tumour indicator or prostate disease.

PSA density: the ratio of PSA value to prostate volume.

PSA doubling time: the time it takes a man's PSA value to double from a new test to the last test.

PSA velocity: the rate of change in a PSA over a period of time.

Prostatitis: inflammation or infection of the prostate.

Radiation: a curative treatment for prostate cancer using X-ray beams of energy for a short duration over the course of several weeks.

Radical prostatectomy: the entire prostate (including the seminal vesicles and the prostatic urethra) are removed to treat prostate cancer; it is a major surgery.

Resectoscope: an instrument used to invade the urethral wall to treat benign hyperplasia of the prostate; inserted into the penis for this purpose while under anesthetic.

Retrograde ejaculation: after transurethral resection sometimes the ejaculate may pass into the bladder opening and not go immediately into the urethra.

Saccule or saccular: tiny sacs filled with fluids; prostate sacs release fluids through tubes or ducts into the urethra.

Semen: a thick whitish mucoid secretion from the testes, prostate, seminal vesicles, Cowper's glands; fluid volume varies from 3-5 ml. and maintains sperm motility and nourishment.

Seminal vesicles: paired glands located at the base of the bladder; similar function as the prostate and empties during ejaculation into the prostatic urethra; provides over 50 % of the ejaculate.

Seminiferous tubules: these are convoluted tubules where the cells in the wall of the tubule undergo cell division (meiosis or spermatogenesis) to produce sex cells or spermatozoa.

Spermatozoa: sperm cells produced by the seminiferous tubules in the testes; used to fertilize the egg normally during sexual intercourse; a component of semen.

Sphincter muscle: a ring of muscles which are present at the orifice from one organ to another - from the bladder to the urethra or as an exit controlling muscle, ex. the anal sphincter.

Stage: refers to the extent of cancer volume or size in the prostate.

Stricture: a blockage of the bladder base caused by scar tissue

Surgical margin: when the pathologist examines the edges of the prostate after surgery; can determine if it is clear or positive for cancer.

Symptom: the condition that accompanies a disease; how a person feels.

Terazosin: sometimes administered to patients with BPH; to relax the muscles of the prostate and bladder and enlarge the urethral opening.

Testis: the male sex organ which produces both sperm cells and testosterone; also refers to as the testicle.

Testosterone: the male sex hormone produced by the testis and primarily responsible for the male secondary sex characteristics.

Therapy: the treatment for a disorder.

Total androgen blockade: combating testosterone with hormones such as LHRH agonists to treat prostate cancer.

TNM Staging: a system for expressing progression of cancer tumours within the prostate and extension beyond.

Transition zone: the region of the prostate surrounding the urethra and common site of BPH; some cancer can arise in this zone.

Transurethral resection: the removal of tissue to treat BPH done through the urethra; method is called transurethral resection of the prostate or TURP.

Ultrasound: sound waves of high frequency used to create a picture within the body like X-rays; echoes like a sonar are recorded in this imaging technique as in a transrectal procedure.

Ureters: the ducts or tubes that take urine from the kidneys to the bladder

Urethra: starts from the neck of the bladder and courses through the penis; necessary to transport urine and semen.

Urologist: specializes in the male and female urinary systems and the reproductive system of males.

Vas deferens: the tubes which lead from the epididymis to the prostate urethra that carry sperm cells; sometimes referred to as ductus deferens.

Vasectomy: the severing of the vas deferens to prevent sperm cells entering the urethra; a form of male sterilization.

Prostate Cancer Support Groups in Canada

The Canadian Prostate Cancer Network (CPCN) whose website is www.cpcn.org keeps an update on Prostate Support Groups across Canada. CPCN is an informative site outlining advances in research and treatment of prostate cancer as one of its goals to the Canadian public and to prostate cancer patients. CPCN is truly "the voice of prostate in Canada" and publishes a Newsletter several times a year. CPCN also published an excellent booklet for patients entitled Prostate Cancer. CPCN also sponsors a National Prostate Cancer Conference annually inviting well known oncologists and urologist from Canada and the United States. The names and contact numbers of support groups change frequently so please refer to the website above for any new updates and where you would be able to find the contact names and telephone number in your province. You may also access the website of The Canadian Prostate Health Council for updates on the list of Support Groups across Canada at: www.canadian-prostate.com. You may also check with Our Voice Magazine, supported by AstraZeneca that lists Support Groups and carries many updates and developments on prostate cancer in Canada. Copies of Our Voice are available to prostate cancer patients. Their address is 400 McGill St., 3 rd Floor, Montreal, Quebec, H2Y 2G1.

Websites

The following are informative Canadian and U.S. websites for prostate and other cancers, cancer research, treatment and health issues.

Recommended Canadian Websites:

www.cancer.ca This is the main Canadian Cancer Society website and other provincial site can be accessed from here.

www.nci.cancer.ca National Cancer Institute of Canada.

www.bc.cancer.ca The Canadian Cancer Society site may also be accessed from here and it is worth checking this site.

www.capca.ca Canadian Association of Provincial Cancer Agencies.

www.bccancer.bc.ca This is not only a B.C. website. Open this site, go to Recommended Links. It lists many Cancer and Health Websites. Click on Cancer Websites to select from the long list...excellent.

www.prostateresearch.ca Canadian Prostate cancer Research Initiative promotes new efforts in prostate cancer research.

www.cuog.org/ The Canadian Oncology Group.

www.cpcn.org/ This is an excellent website and it is the Canadian Prostate Cancer Network linking to Canadian research, support groups, magazines and newsletters.

www.phac-aspc.gc.ca/publicat/prccc-relccc/chap_3_e.html Progress Report on Cancer Control in Canada.

www.cancercontrol.org Canadian Strategy for Cancer Control.

www.canadian-health-network.ca/ Many useful topics on a variety of health issues, disease prevention and more.

www.prostatecancer.ca Prostate Cancer Research Foundation of Canada.

www.canadian-prostate.com Canadian Prostate Health Council – updates, projects and more....

www.prostateline.com Prostate Line.

www.healthgate.com Health, wellness and biomedical information.

www.healing.bc.ca The Centre for Integrated Healing. The Centre promotes complementary care for cancer patients and bridges the gap between conventional and alternative therapies.

www.cmshc.org Canadian Male Sexual Health Council.

Recommended U.S. Websites:

www.cancer.org/ The American Cancer Society main page – excellent resources.

http://cancer.gov/search/pubmed An excellent resource on research and abstracts from hundreds of prostate and other cancer sites and much more. The NCI links to PubMed, then for example, search for prostate cancer.

www.drcatalona.com/links.asp Urological Research Foundation; it's an excellent site with research articles and Dr. Catalona's articles on prostate cancer and treatment options.

www.bcm.edu/cancercenter/links.htm The Cancer Center with links to websites.

www.prostate-cancer.org Prostate Cancer Research Institute; an update on many emerging treatment options and more.

www.mskcc.org/mskcc/html/11570.cfm Memorial Sloan-Kettering Cancer Center's website includes information about herbs, phytochemicals and other products on alternative healing practices.

www.nci.nih.gov National Cancer Institute provides information on cancer screening, diagnosis and treatment.

www.cancer.gov National Cancer Institute.

www.niddk.nih.gov National Institute of Diabetes and digestive and Kidney Diseases.

www.impotence.org provides information on erectile dysfunction.

www.incontinence.org provides information on urinary incontinence.

www.prostate.urol.jhu/prostate/cancer The Brady Urological Institute provides research materials.

www.ustoo.com U.S. Prostate Support Group serves support groups and provides useful information

www.nlm.nih.gov to access scientific articles.

www.quackwatch.org/ A guide to quackery, health fraud, and intelligent decisions.

www.fhcrc.org The Hutchison Cancer Research Center in Seattle, Washington State. Presents epidemiological studies and patient information on prostate cancer.

References

Chapter 1

Bochum, S *et al.* "Confirmation of the Prostate Cancer Susceptibility Locus HPCX in set of 104 German Prostate Cancer Families." *PubMed*, June 2002, www.ncbi.nlm.nih.gov/.

Cheng, Iona *et al.* "Comparison of Prostate Specific Antigen and Hormone Levels among Men in Singapore and the United States." *Cancer Epidemiology Biomarkers & Prevention.* Vol. 14, July 2005: 1692 – 1696.

Farnsworth, E & Ablin, R. *The Prostate as an Endocrine Gland.* CRC Press, 1990.

Gann, Peter *et al.* "Prospective study of Sex Hormone Levels and Risk of Prostate Cancer." *Journal of the National Cancer Institute.* Vol. 88, No. 16, August, 1996: 1118 – 1126.

Mader, Sylvia. *Inquiry Into Life.* McGraw Hill Higher Education, 10th Edition, New York, 2003.

Perinchery, G *et al.* "Deletion of Y-chromosome specific genes in human prostate cancer." *PubMed,* April, 2000, www.ncbi.nlm.nih.gov/.

Rous, Stephen, N. *The Prostate Book - Sound Advice on Symptoms and Treatment.* W.W. Norton & Co., New York, 2001.

Scardino, Peter & Kelman, Judith. *The Prostate Book.* Avery (Penguin Group) Publication, New York, 2005.

Walsh, Patrick & Worthington, Janet. *Guide to Surviving Prostate Cancer.* Warner Books, New York, 2001.

Zheng, S. L *et al.* "Evidence for a Prostate Cancer Linkage to Chromosome 20 in 159 Hereditary Prostate Cancer Families." *PubMed,* May 2001. www.ncbi.nlm.nih.gov/.

Chapter 2

Bochum, S. et al. "Confirmation of the Prostate Cancer Susceptibility Locus HPCX in set of 104 German Prostate Cancer Families." *PubMed,* June 2002, www.ncbi.nlm.nih.gov/.

Canadian Cancer Society. "Working Together to Understand the Genetics of Prostate Cancer." *PROGRESS Against Cancer.* Vol. 48, No.1, March 1994.

Downing, Sean *et al.* "Alterations of p53 are common in Early Stage Prostate Cancer." *The Canadian Journal of Urology,* Vol. 10, No. 4, August, 2003: 1924 - 1933.

De Kok, Jacques, *et al.* "DD3PCA3, A Very Sensitive and Specific Marker to Detect Prostate Cancer." *Cancer Research,* May 1, 2002.

Fradet, Yves et al. "uPM3, A New Molecular Urine Test for the Detection of Prostate Cancer." *Urology,* Vol. 64, No. 2, August, 2004: 311 - 316.

Garnick, Marc B. "The Dilemmas of Prostate Cancer." *Scientific American,* April 1994.

Garnick, Marc B & Fair, William R. "Combating Prostate Cancer." *Scientific American,* Dec. 1998 & Quarterly Issue, "Men". July, 1999.

Hessels, Daphne *et al.* "DD3PCA3 - based Molecular Urine Analysis for Diagnosis of Prostate Cancer." *European Urology,* Vol. 44, May 2003: 8 - 19.

Perinchery, G *et al.* "Deletion of Y-chromosome Specific Genes in Human Prostate Cancer." *PubMed,* April, 2000, www.ncbi.nlm.nih.gov/.

Scientific American Special Issue. "What You Need To Know About Cancer." September, 1996.

Slager, S.L. "Confirmation of Linkage of Prostate Cancer Aggressiveness with Chromosome 19 q." March 2003, *PubMed,* www.ncbi.nlm.nih/.

Xu, J et al. "Linkage of Prostate Cancer Susceptibility Loci to Chromosome 1." *PubMed,* April, 2001, www.ncbi.nlm.gov/.

Zhang, K.Q *et al.* "Genetics of Prostate Cancer." January, 2003, *PubMed,* www.ncbi.nlm.nih.gov/.

Zheng, S.L. *et al.* "Evidence for a Prostate Cancer Linkage to Chromosome 20 in 159 Hereditary Prostate Cancer Families." *PubMed,* May 2001, www.ncbi.nlm.nih.gov/.

"Genetics of Prostate Cancer." *National Cancer Institute,* March 2005. www.cancer.gov/cancertopics/pdq/genetics/prostate/.

"Prostate Cancer Genetic Therapy." Prostate Cancer Research Institute, Summer 2000, www.prostate-cancer.org/education/genetics.

"Gene therapy for prostate cancer." *BBC News,* June 2001, www.bbc.co.uk.

"Emory Scientists Find New Prostate Cancer Suppressor Gene." March 22, 2005, www.sciencedaily.com/.

"Tumour Suppressor Genes: p53." Prostate Cancer Research Institute. Lecture in 1994, www.prostate-cancer.org/education/genetics.

Chapter 3

Bent, Stephen *et al.* "Saw Palmetto for Benign Prostate Hyperplasia." *New England Journal of Medicine,* Vol. 354, No. 6, February 9, 2006: 557 – 566.

Catalona, William. "Drug Therapy: Management of Prostate Cancer." *New England Journal of Medicine,* October 13, 1994: 996 - 1004.

De la Rosette, J.J. *et al.* "Current Status of Thermotherapy of the Prostate." *The Journal of Urology,* Vol. 157 (2), February 1997: 430 - 438.

Gormley, Glenn J. "The Effect of Finasteride in Men with Benign Prostatic Hyperplasia." *New England J. Medicine,* October 22, 1992: 1185 - 1191.

Gray, Ross *et al.* "Restoring Sexual Function in Prostate Cancer Patients: an Innovative Approach." *The Canadian Journal of Urology, 11* (3), June 2004: 2285 - 2289.

Hoffman, Richard *et al.* "Laser Versus Transurethral Resection for Treating Benign Prostatic Obstruction." *The Journal of Urology,* Vol. 169 (1), January 2003: 210 - 215.

Larson, Thayne *et al.* "Detailed Interstitial Temperature Mapping During Treatment with a Novel Transurethral Microwave Thermoablation System in Patients with Benign Prostatic Hyperplasia." *The Journal of Urology,* Vol. 159 (1), January 1998: 258 - 264.

Martin, William & Scardino, Peter. *My Prostate and Me.* Cardell & Davies, N.Y., 1994.

Our Voice - Living with Prostate Cancer in Canada, Spring, Summer, Fall & Winter Issues, 1998 - 2004.

Rous, Stephen. *The Prostate Book – Sound Advice on Symptoms and Treatment.* W.W. Norton & Co., New York, 2001.

Scardino, Peter & Kelman, Judith. *The Prostate Book.* Avery (Penguin Group) Publication, New York, 2005.

Sherar, Michael et al. "Interstitial Microwave Thermal Therapy for Prostate Cancer: Method of Treatment and Results of Phase I/II Trial." *The J. Urology,* Vol. 166 (5), November 2001: 1707 - 1714.

So, Alan. "Prostate Cancer Prevention?" *Our Voice,* Vol. 1, No. 4, January 2006: p. 14.

The Johns Hopkins Medical Letter. "Is Proscar Right for You?" Vol. 4, Issue 7, September 1992.

The Johns Hopkins Medical Letter. "Enlarged Prostate: Evaluating Your Options." Vol.7, Issue 2, April 1995.

Thompson, Ian *et al.* "The Influence of Finasteride on the Development of Prostate Cancer." *New England Journal of Medicine,* Vol. 349, No. 3, July 17, 2003: 215 - 224.

Tooher, Rebecca *et al.* "A Systematic Review of Holium Laser Prostatectomy for Benign Prostatic Hyperplasia." *The Journal of Urology,* Vol. 171 (5), May 2004: 1773 - 1781.

Walsh, Patrick & Worthington, Janet. *Guide to Surviving Prostate Cancer.* Warner Books, New York, 2001.

Wilt, Timothy *et al.* "Saw Palmetto Extracts for Treatment of Benign Prostatic Hyperplasia." *Journal of the American Medical Association,* Vol. 280, No. 18, November 1998: 1604 – 1609.

"BPH: Treatment: International Prostate Symptoms Score." The Prostate Centre, Vancouver General Hospital. www.prostatecentre.com.

"International Prostate Symptoms Score." *Patient Plus,* August 2005. www.patient.co.uk.

Chapter 4

Augustsson, Katarina *et al.* "A Prospective Study of Intake of Fish and Marine Fatty Acids and Prostate Cancer." *Cancer Epidemiology Biomarkers & Prevention.* Vol. 12, January 2003: 64 – 67.

Bodiwala, D *et al.* "Prostate Cancer Risk and Exposure to Ultraviolet Radiation: Further Support for the Protection of Sunlight." *PubMed,* 2003. www.ncbi.nlm.nih.gov/.

Barber, N *et al.* "Dietary Supplementation with oral Lycopene in Men with Histological proven Adenocarcinoma." *Abstract Uroweb,* March 17, 2005. www.uroweb.nl/index.

Bairati, Isabelle *et al.* "Dietary Fat and Advanced Prostate Cancer." *The Journal of Urology*, Vol. 159 (4), April 1998: 1271 - 1275.

Bunker, Clareann *et al.* "High Prevalence of Screening-detected Prostate Cancer among Afro-Caribbean – The Tobago Prostate Cancer Survey." *Cancer Epidemiology Biomarkers & Prevention,* Vol. 11, August 2002: 726 – 729.

Bratt, Ola. "Hereditary Prostate Cancer." *The Journal of Urology,* Vol. 163 (3), September 2002: 906 – 913.

Calle, Eugenia *et al.* "Overweight, Obesity, and Mortality from Cancer in a Prospectively Studied Cohort of U.S. Adults." *New England Journal of Medicine,* Vol. 348, No. 17, April 2003: 1625 – 1638.

Canadian Cancer Society. "Prostate Cancer Resources." Memo, March 28, 1995.

Canadian Cancer Society. *Canadian Cancer Statistics , 1997, 1998, 2005 & 2006.* National Cancer Institute of Canada, Toronto.

Carroll, Peter. "Obesity and Prostate Cancer." The Prostate Cancer Symposium reported in *Insights Newsletter.* Prostate Cancer Research Institute, Vol. 9, No. 2, May 2006: 1-12.

Catalona, William. "Drug Therapy: Management of Prostate Cancer." *New England Journal of Medicine,* October 13, 1994: 996 – 1004.

Cheng, Iona *et al.* "Comparison of Prostate Specific Antigen and Hormone Levels among Men in Singapore and the United States." *Cancer Epidemiology Biomarkers & Prevention.* Vol. 14, July 2005: 1692 – 1696.

Downing, Sean *et al.* "Alterations of p53 are common in early stage prostate cancer." *The Canadian Journal of Urology,* Vol. 10, No. 4, August 2003: 1924 – 1933.

Fleshner, Neil. "Dietary Factors in Slowing the Development of Prostate Cancer." *Canadian Prostate Cancer Network* (CD Rom), National Conference, Calgary, 2004.

Garnick, Mark & Fair, William. "Combating Prostate Cancer." *Scientific American,* Dec. 1998 & Quarterly Issue: "Men." July 1999.

Gapstur, Susan *et al.* "Serum Androgen Concentrations in Young Men: A Longitudinal Analysis of Associations with Age, Obesity, and Race. The CARDIA Male Hormone study." *Cancer Epidemiology Biomarkers & Prevention.* Vol. 11, October 2002: 1041 – 1047.

Giovannucci, Edward *et al.* "A Prospective Cohort Study of Vasectomy and Prostate Cancer in US Men." *Journal of the American Medical Association,* Vol. 269, No. 7, February 17, 1993: 873 - 877.

Giovannucci, E.L *et al.* "A Prospective Study of Physical Activity and Incident and Fatal Prostate Cancer." *PubMed,* May 9, 2005.

Grimm, Peter (Editor) *et al. The Prostate Cancer Treatment Book.* McGraw-Hill, New York, 2003.

Heber, David. "Linkage between Obesity and Prostate Cancer." *Insights Newslstter,* Prostate Cancer Research Institute, Vol. 7. No. 1, May 2004.

Hemminki, Kari "Familial association of prostate cancer with other cancers in the Swedish Family -Cancer Database." *Wiley InterScience,* Vol. 65, Issue 2, June 2005.

HOPE Trial. "Effects of Long-term Vitamin E Supplements on Cardiovascular Events and Cancer." *Journal of the American Medical Association,* Vol. 293, No. 11, March 16, 2005: 1338 - 1347.

I-Min Lee *et al.* "Vitamin E in the Primary Prevention of Cardiovascular Disease and Cancer." *Journal of the American Medical Association,* Vol. 294 (1), July 6, 2005: 56 - 65.

Kirchhoff, Tomas *et al.* "BRCA Mutations and Risk of Prostate Cancer in Ashkenazi Jews." *Clinical Cancer Research,* Vol. 10, May 2004: 2918 – 2921.

Kirsh, Victoria et al. "A Prospective Study of Lycopene and Tomato product Intake and Risk of Prostate Cancer." *Cancer Epidemiology Biomarkers & Prevention,* Vol. 15, January 2006: 92 – 98.

Leichtenstein, Paul *et al.* "Environmental and Heritable Factors in the Causation of Cancer - Analyses of Cohorts of Twins from Sweden, Denmark and Finland." *New England of J. Medicine,* Vol. 343, No. 2, July 13, 2000: 78 - 85.

Lu, Qing-Yi *et al.* "Inverse Associations between Plasma Lycopene and Other Carotenoids and Prostate Cancer." *Cancer Epidemiology Biomarkers & Prevention.* Vol. 10, July 2001: 749 – 756.

Marks, Sheldon. *Prostate & Cancer. A Family Guide to Diagnosis, Treatment & Survival.* Fisher Books, Arizona, 1995.

Marks, L.S. "Prostate cancer in native Japanese and Japanese -American men: effects of dietary differences on prostatic tissue." *PubMed,* 2004, www.ncbi.nlm.nih.gov/.

Meikle, Wayne A. & Smith, Joseph A. "Epidemiology of Prostate Cancer." *Urologic Clinics of North America,* W.B. Saunders, Phil., November 1990.

McKenzie, D.C. "The Importance of Exercise in Prostate Cancer Therapy." Lecture at the Vancouver Prostate Support & Awareness Group, November 2005.

Nagata, Chisato *et al.* "Effect of Soymilk Consumption on Serum Estrogen and Androgen Concentrations in Japanese Men." *Cancer Epidemiology Biomarkers & Prevention.* Vol. 10, March 2001: 179 – 184.

Nam, Robert *et al.* "Serum Insulin-Like Growth Factor-1 Levels and Prostatic Intraepithelial Neoplasia: A Clue to the Relationship between IGF-1 Physiology and Prostate Cancer Risk." *Cancer Epidemiology Biomarkers & Prevention.* Vol.14 (5), May 2005: 1270 – 1273.

Oakley- Girvan, Ingrid *et al.* "Risk of Early-Onset Prostate Cancer in Relation to Germ Line Polymorphisms of Vitamin D Receptor." *Cancer Epidemiology Biomarkers & Prevention.* Vol.13 (8), August 2004: 1325 – 1330.

Ornish, Dean *et al.* "Intensive Lifestyle Changes May Affect Prostate Cancer." *The Journal of Urology,* Vol. 174 (3), September 2005: 1065 – 1070.

Ornish, Dean *et al.* "Intensive Lifestyle Changes for Reversal of Coronary Heart Disease." *JAMA,* Vol. 23, No. 23, December 16, 1998: 2001 -

Our Voice – Living with Prostate Cancer. Vols. 1 & 2, Nos. 1 & 2, Summer & Fall 2005.

Pickles, Tom *et al.* "The Changing Face of Prostate Cancer in British Columbia 1988 - 2000." *The Canadian Journal of Urology,* 9 (3), June 2002: 1551 - 1557.

Platz, Elizabeth *et al.* "Statins May halve Advanced Prostate Cancer." *Health Day,* www.healthyday.com, June, 2005.

Rodriguez, Carmen *et al.* "Meat Consumption among Black and White Men and Risk of Prostate Cancer in the Cancer Prevention Study 11 Nutrition Cohort." *Cancer Epidemiology Biomarkers & Prevention,* Vol. 15, February 2006: 211 – 216.

Salvatore, Steve. "Finnish Study of Men Taking Vitamin E." April 1998, www.cnn.com/health/.

Scardino, Peter & Kelman, Judith. *The Prostate Book.* Avery (Penguin Group) Publication, New York, 2005.

Severi, Gianluca *et al.* "Circulating Steroid Hormones and the Risk of Prostate Cancer." *Cancer Epidemiology Biomarkers & Prevention,* Vol. 15, January 2006: 86 – 91.

Sgambato, A *et al.* "Resveratrol, a Natural Phenolic Compound, Inhibits Cell Proliferation and Prevents Oxidative DNA Damage." September 2001, *PubMed,* www.ncbi.nlm.nih.gov/.

Stamm, Jason & Ornstein, Deborah. "The Role of Statins in Cancer Prevention and Treatment." *Oncology,* Vol. 19, No. 6, May 2005: 729 - 745.

Stanford, Janet *et al.* "A Glass of Red Wine a Day May Keep Prostate Cancer Away." Hutchison Cancer Research Center, September 2004. www.fhcrc.org.

Stanford, Janet *et al.* "Long-term Smoking Doubles the Risk of More Aggressive Prostate Cancer in Middle-aged Men." Hutchison Cancer Research Center, July 2003. www.fhcrc.org.

Strum, Stephen & Pogliano, Donna. *A Primer on Prostate Cancer – The Empowered Patient Guide.* The Life Extension Foundation, Florida, 2005.

Tammela, T *et al.* "Preliminary Results from the Third Round of the Finnish Prostate Cancer Screening Trial." *Abstract Uroweb,* March 18, 2005. www.uroweb.nl/index.

Thompson, Ian *et al.* "Prevalence of Prostate Cancer among Men with a Prostate-Specific Antigen Level of less than or equal to 4.0 ng/ml." *New England Journal of Medicine,* Vol. 350, No. 22, May 27, 2004: 2239 - 2246

Verhage, B.A *et al.* "Site-specific Familial Aggregation of Prostate Cancer." *Pub Med.* 2004, www.ncbi.nlm.nih.gov/.

Walsh, P & A.W. Partin. "Family History Facilitates the Early Diagnosis of Prostate Cancer." *PubMed,* 1997. www.ncbi.nlm.nih.gov/.

Walsh, Patrick & Worthington, Janet. *Guide to Surviving Prostate Cancer.* Warner Books, New York, 2001.

Wen-Hsiang, Lee *et al.* "Cytidine Methylation of Regulatory Sequences class - near Gluthathione S-transferase Gene accompanies Human Prostatic Carcinogenesis." Proceedings of the National Academy of Science, November 1994.

Wiens, Kristin *et al.* The Prostate Education & Research Centre (The Prostate Centre), *Vancouver General Hospital. Nutrition Page,* 2005.

Zeegers, M.P. *et al.* "Physical Activity and the Risk of Prostate Cancer in the Netherlands Cohort Study, Results after 9.3 years of follow-up." *PubMed,* June 2005.

Vancouver Prostate & Awareness Support Group. Notes from Lectures by Urologists, Oncologists, Epidemiologists & Nutritionists, 2003 – 2005.

"High Cholesterol Levels Accelerate the Growth of Prostate Cancer." Children's Hospital, Boston. March 27, 2005. www.sciencedaily.com.

"Heart Attack Prevention." John Hopkins Health After 50, 2005. www.hopkinsafter50.com.

Chapter 5

Andriole, Gerald. Editorial: "Prostate Specific Antigen Based Prostate Cancer Screening: Accumulating Evidence of Efficacy but Persistent Uncertainty." *The Journal of Urology,* Vol. 174, August 2005: 413 - 414.

Bader, A *et al.* "Prostate Cancer with a Low PSA - A Harmless Tumor?" *Abstract Uroweb*, March 17, 2005. www.uroweb.nl/index.

Bektic, L *et al.* "Correlation between Gleason Score of Needle Biopsies and Score of Radical Prostatectomy: 12 Years Experience." *Abstract Uroweb,* March 19, 2005. www.uroweb.org/index.

B.C. Cancer Agency. "Prostate –Predisposing Factors & Prevention". Report from Drs. Gallagher & Fleshner, www.bccancer.bc.ca.

Carter, H.B *et al.* "Recommended Prostate-specific Antigen Testing Intervals for Detection of Curable Prostate Cancer." *Journal of the American Medical Association*, Vol. 277, No. 18, May 14, 1997:1456 - 1460.

Carter, Ballentine, H. "Prostate Cancers in Men with low PSA Levels - Must We Find them?" *New England Journal of Medicine,* Vol. 350, No. 22, May 27, 2004: 2292 - 2294.

Catalona, William *et al.* "Use of the Percentage of Free Prostate-Specific Antigen to Enhance Differentiation of Prostate Cancer From Benign Prostatic Disease." *Journal of the American Medical Association,* Vol. 279, No. 19, May 20, 1998: 1542 - 1547.

Catalona, William *et al*. "Serum Pro-PSA Preferentially Detects Aggressive Prostate Cancer in Men with 2 to 4 ng/ml Prostate Specific Antigen." *The Journal of Urology,* Vol. 171, (6), June 2004: 2239 - 2244.

Catalona, W. "Markers for Prostate Cancer: What's New?" Urological Research Foundation, www.drcatalona.com/quest/quest. Fall 2002.

Centre for Health Services. "Prostate Specific Antigen in early Detection of Prostate Cancer." University of B.C., September 1993.

Crawford, E.D. *et al*. "The Effects of Digital Rectal Examination on Prostate Specific Antigen Levels." *Journal of the American Medical Association,* Vol. 267, No. 16, April 22, 1992: 2227 - 2228.

D'Amico, Anthony *et al*. "Preoperative PSA Velocity and Risk of Death from Prostate Cancer after Radical Prostatectomy." *New England Journal of Medicine,* Vol. 351, No. 2, July 8, 2004: 125 - 135.

Editorial. "Early Stage of Prostate Cancer - Do we have a problem with Over-detection and Over-treatment or both?" *The Journal of Urology*, Vol. 173, No. 4, April 2005: 1061 - 1062.

Etzioni, Ruth *et al*. "Prostate-Specific Antigen and Free Prostate-Specific Antigen in the Early Detection of Prostate Cancer: Do Combination Tests Improve Detection?" *Cancer Epidemiology Biomarkers & Prevention*. Vol. 13 (10), October 2004: 1640-1645.

Fradet, Yves *et al*. "uPM3, A New Molecular Urine Test for the Detection of Prostate Cancer." *Urology,* Vol.64, No.2, August 2004:311 - 316

Frauscher, Ferdinand *et al*. "Comparison of Contrast Enhanced Doppler Targeted Biopsy with Conventional Systematic Biopsy: Impact on prostate Detection." *The Journal of Urology*, Vol. 167 (4), April, 2002: 1648 - 1652.

Gleave, Martin E. "The Early Detection of Prostate Cancer." *B.C. Medical Journal*, June 6, 1994.

Gleave, Martin. "Prostate Cancer Detection, Treatment, and Research." *Canadian Prostate Cancer Network* (CD Rom), National Conference, 2004.

Goldenberg, Larry S & Thompson, Ian. *Prostate Cancer. Intelligent Patient Guide*, Vancouver, 2001.

Harisinghani, Mukesh *et al*. "Noninvasive Detection of Clinically Occult Lymph-Node Metastases in Prostate Cancer." *New England Journal of Medicine,* Vol. 348, No. 25, June 19, 2003: 2491 - 2499.

Hugosson, Jonas *et al*. "Prostate Specific Antigen Based Biennial Screening is Sufficient to Detect Almost All Prostate Cancers while still Curable." *The Journal of Urology*, Vol. 169, May 2003: 1720 - 1723.

Kopek, Jacek *et al.* "Screening with Prostate Specific Antigen and Metastatic Prostate Cancer Risk: A Population Based Case-Controlled Study." *The Journal of Urology,* Vol. 174 (2), August 2005: 475 - 499.

Lein, Michael *et al.* "A Multicenter Clinical Trial on the Use of (-5,-7) Pro Prostate Specific Antigen." *The Journal of Urology,* Vol. 174 (6), December 2005: 2150 - 2153.

Marks, Sheldon. *Prostate Cancer. A Family Guide to Diagnosis, Treatment & Survival.* Fischer Books, Arizona, 1995.

McDermed, Jonathan. "Using PSA Intelligently to Manage Prostate Cancer." *PCRI Insights Newsletter,* Vol. 8, No. 3, August 2005: 6 – 10.

Nam, Robert *et al.* "A Novel Serum Marker, Total Prostate Secretory Protein of 94 Amino Acids, Improves Prostate Cancer Detection and Helps Identify High Grade Cancers at Diagnosis." *The Journal of Urology,* Vol. 175, Issue 4, April 2006: 1291-1297.

Oesterling, Joseph E *et al.* "Serum Prostate Specific Antigen in a Community-Based Population of Healthy Men. Establishment of Age Specific Ranges." *Journal of the American Medical Association,* Vol. 270, No. 7, August 18, 1993: 860 - 864.

Paul, Barbara *et al.* "Detection of Prostate Cancer with a Blood-Based Assay for Early Prostate Cancer." *Cancer Research,* May 15, 2005. http://cancerre.aacrjournals.org.

Pickles, Tom. "Prostate Specific Antigen -PSA." B. C. Cancer Agency Library Files, April 1993.

Phillip, J *et al.* "Is a Digital Rectal Exam necessary in the diagnosis and clinical staging of early prostate cancer?" *British Journal Urology International,* May 2005. www.ncbi.nlm.nih.gov/.

Punglia, Rinaa *et al.* "Effect of Verification on Screening for Prostate Cancer by Management of PSA." *New England Journal of Medicine,* Vol. 349, No. 4, July 24, 2003: 335 - 341.

Reichel, Jules on Dr. Dan Vick's research: "One Man to Another – The Pathology Point of View." Fall 2005, www.catalona.com/quest.

Scardino, Peter & Kelman, Judith. *The Prostate Book.* Avery (Penguin Group) Publication, New York, 2005.

Shibata, Atsuko *et al.* "Serum Levels of Prostate- Specific Antigen among Japanese-American and Native Japanese Men." *Journal of the National Cancer Institute.* Vol. 89, No. 22, November 1997: 1716 – 1720.

So, Alan *et al.* "Prostate Specific Antigen: An Update Review." *The Canadian Journal of Urology,* Vol. 10, No. 6, December 2003: 2040 - 2050.

Strum, Stephen. "What Every Doctor Who Treats Male Patients Should Know." Prostate Cancer Research Institute, *Insights Newsletter,* Vol. 8, No. 2, May 2005.

Sved, Paul *et al.* "Limitations of Biopsy Gleason Grade: Implications for Counseling Patients with Biopsy Gleason Score 6 Prostate Cancer." *The Journal of Urology,* Vol. 172, July 2004: 98 - 102.

Tammela, T *et al.* "Preliminary Results from the Third Round of the Finnish Prostate Cancer Screening Trial." *Abstract Uroweb,* March 18, 2005. www.uroweb.nl/index.

Tariel, E *et al.* "The Effect of Bicycle Riding on PSA." *Abstract Uroweb,* March 18, 2005. www.uroweb.ni/index.

The Johns Hopkins Medical Letter. "New discovery may improve the value of PSA." Vol. 7, Issue 11, January 1996.

Thompson, Ian *et al.* "Prevalence of Prostate Cancer among Men with a Prostate-Specific Antigen Level of less than or equal to 4.0 ng/ml." *New England Journal of Medicine,* Vol. 350, No. 22, May 27, 2004: 2239 – 2246.

Thompson, Ian *et al.* "Operating Characteristics of Prostate-Specific Antigen in Men with an Initial PSA level of 3.0 ng/ml or Lower." *Journal of the American Medical Association,* Vol. 294, No. 1, July 2005: 66 - 70.

Walsh, Patrick & Worthington, Janet. *Guide to Surviving Prostate Cancer.* Warner Books, New York, 2001.

Wang, Xiaoju *et al.* "Autoantibody Signatures in Prostate Cancer." *New England Journal of Medicine,* Vol. 353, No. 12, September 2005: 1224-1235.

"Canadian Cancer Society- funded study adds important information to early PSA Screening issue." *Canadian Cancer Society,* 2005 - www.cancer.ca.

Vancouver Prostate & Awareness Support Group. Notes from Lectures by Urologists & Oncologists, 2003 - 2005.

"The Truth about PSA Testing." September 15, 2004 - Canadian Prostate Cancer Network - www.cpcn.org/archives/.

"The Diagnosis." Prostateinfo.com., March 2003, www.prostateinfo.com/patient/diagnosis.

Dr. Catalona's Website (www.catalona.com/quest/) "Lowering PSA Threshold to 2.6 is Sound Practice." September 2002.

Dr. Catalona's Website (www.catalona.com/quest/) "Tumor Volume and Prostate Cancer." Winter 2003.

"PSA Screening - 6 Positions of Other Medical Organizations on Screening for Prostate Cancer with PSA." September 2003, B.C. Cancer Agency. www.bccancer.bc.ca.

Chapter 6

Arbelaez Arango, S *et al.* "Gleason Score 3+4 and 4+3 T1C Prostate Cancer; Clinical and Histopathological Differences Found in 117 Radical Prostatectomies." *Abstract Uroweb,* March 19, 2005. www.uroweb.org/index.

Austenfeld, Mark & Davis, Bradley. "New Concepts in the Treatment of Stage D1 Adenocarcinoma of the Prostate." *The Urologic Clinics of North America,* W.B. Saunders, Philadelphia, November 1990.

Beltic, L et al. "Correlation between Gleason Score of Needle Biopsy and Score of Radical Prostatectomy: 12 Years Experience." *Abstract Uroweb,* March 19, 2005. www.uroweb.org/.

Catalona, William. "Drug Therapy: Management of Prostate Cancer." *New England Journal of Medicine,* October 13, 1994: 996 – 1004.

Eskicorapci, S *et al.* "Validation of 2001 Partin Tables in Turkey: A Multicenter Study." *Abstract Uroweb,* March 19, 2005. www.uroweb.org/index.

Fallon, Bernard & Williams, Richard. "Current Options in the Management of Clinical Stage C Prostatic Carcinoma." *The Urologic Clinics of North America,* W.B. Saunders, Philadelphia, November 1990.

Fleming, Craig *et al.* "A Decision of Alternative Treatment Strategies for Clinically Localized Cancer." *Journal of the American Medical Association,* Vol. 269, No. 20, 26 May, 1993: 2650 - 2658.

Freedland, Stephen *et al.* "The Prostatic Specific Antigen Era is Alive and Well: Prostatic Specific Antigen and Biochemical Progression Following Radical Prostatectomy." *The Journal of Urology,* Vol. 174 (4), October 2005: 1276-1281.

Gleave, Martin *et al.* "Biochemical and Pathological Effects of 8 Months of Neoadjuvant Androgen Withdrawal Therapy before Radical Prostatectomy in Patients with Clinically Confined Prostate Cancer." *The Journal of Urology,* Vol. 155 (1), January 1996: 213 – 219.

Goldenberg, Larry & Thompson, Ian. *Prostate Cancer. Intelligent Patient Guide,* Vancouver, 2001.

Kaisary, Amir *et al. Textbook of Prostate Cancer - Pathology, Diagnosis, Treatment.* Martin Dunitz Ltd., 1999.

Kantoff, Philip *et al. Prostate Cancer Principles and Practice.* Lippincott Williams & Wilkins, 2002.

Lange, Paul. *Prostate Cancer for Dummies.* Wiley Publishing, Inc., New York, 2003.

Lewis, James & Berger, Roy. *Guidelines for Surviving Prostate Cancer.* Health Education Literary Publication, New York, 1997.

Pound, Charles *et al*. "Natural History of Progression after PSA Elevation Following Radical Prostatectomy." *Journal of the American Medical Association,* Vol. 281, No. 17, May 5, 1999: 1591 - 1597.

Ross, P.L *et al*. "Comparisons of Nomograms and Urologists' Predictions in Prostate Cancer." *PubMed,* May 2002, www.ncbi.nlm.nih.gov/.

Scardino, Peter & Kelman, Judith. *The Prostate Book.* Avery (Penguin Group) Publication, New York, 2005.

Tisman, Glenn. "Using Nomograms to Predict Pathological Stage Treatment Outcome for Patients with Prostate Cancer." *PCRI Insights,* November 2005.

Walsh, Patrick & Worthington, Janet. *Guide to Surviving Prostate Cancer.* Warner Books, New York, 2001.

Warner, John A. "The Management of Prostate Cancer." *B.C. Medical Journal,* 6 June, 1994.

Zinner, Norman R. *Everyone's Guide to Cancer Therapy.* Sommerville House Publication, Toronto, 1992.

"Staging Systems." Oncology Channel, April 2005, www.oncologychannel.com/prostatecancer.

Chapter 7

Albertsen, Peter *et al*. "Competing Risk Analysis of Men Aged 55 to 74 Years at Diagnosis Managed Conservatively for Clinically Localized Prostate Cancer." *Journal of the America Medical Association,* Vol. 280, No. 11, September 16, 1998: 975 - 980.

Bahn, Duke. "Cryosurgery in the Treatment of Prostate Cancer." Crittenton Hospital, Rochester, Michigan, February 2005, www.cancernews.com.

Bahn, Duke *et al* "Cryoablation of the Prostate." Prostate Cancer Research Institute, February 2005 - www.prostate-cancer.org.

Bahn, Duke. "Cryotherapy." Prostate Institute of America, www.pioa.org, 2003.

Blana, A *et al*. "High Intensity Focused Ultrasound for the Treatment of Localized Prostate Cancer: 5-year experience." *PubMed,* 2004. www.ncbi.nlm.nih.gov/.

Cadeddu, Jeffery *et al*. "Long-term Results of Radiation Therapy for Prostate Cancer Recurrence following Radical Prostatectomy." *The Journal of Urology,* Vol. 159 (1), January 1998: 173 – 177.

Chinn, Douglas. "Transrectal HIFU: The Next Generation?" Prostate Cancer Research Institute, *Insights Newsletter,* Vol. 8, No. 1, February 2004.

Freedland, Stephen *et al*. "Obesity and Capsular Incision at the time of Open Retropubic Radical Prostatectomy." *The Journal of Urology,* Vol. 174 (5), November 2005: 1798 – 1801.

Geary, Stewart *et al.* "Nerve Sparing Radical Prostatectomy: A Different View." *The Journal of Urology,* Vol. 154, No. 1 July, 1995: 145 - 149.

Gelet, A et al. "Local Control of Prostate Cancer by Transrectal High Intensity Focused Ultrasound Therapy: Preliminary Results." *The Journal of Urology,* Vol. 161 (1), January 1999: 156 - 162.

Gleave, Martin E. *et al.* "Randomized Comparative Study of 3 versus 8- Month Neoadjuvant Hormonal Therapy before Radical Prostatectomy: Biochemical and Pathological Effects." *The Journal of Urology,* Vol. 166 (2), August 2001: 500 - 507.

Gleave, Martin *et al.* "Biochemical and Pathological Effects of 8 Months of Neoadjuvant Androgen Withdrawal Therapy before Radical Prostatectomy in patients with Clinically Confined Prostate Cancer." *The Journal of Urology,* Vol. 155 (1), January 1996: 213- 219.

Gleave, Martin. "Prostate Cancer Detection, Treatment, and Research." *Canadian Prostate Cancer Network* (CD Rom), National Conference, 2004.

Goldenberg, Larry & Thompson, Ian. *Prostate Cancer. Intelligent Patient Guide,* Vancouver, 2001.

Kipper, S. "Update on ProstaScint, CT & MRI Fusion as Diagnostic Tools." *Prostate Cancer Research Institute,* Vol. 6, No. 3, August 2003.

Lu-Yao, Grace *et al.* "An Assessment of Radical Prostatectomy. Time Trends, Geographical Variation, and Outcomes. The Prostate Pattern Outcome Research." *Journal of the American Medical Association,* May 26, 1993: 2633 - 2641.

Martin, William & Scardino, Peter. *My prostate and Me.* Cardell & Davies, New York, 1994.

Neufert, Debbie. "Robotic Cancer Surgery at CSTAR a Canadian first." *Hospital News.* September 2004. www.hospitalnews.com/modules/

Pickles, Tom *et al.* "Technology review: High-Intensity Focused Ultrasound for Prostate Cancer." *The Canadian Journal of Urology,* 12(2), April 2005: 2593 - 2597.

Poissonnier, L *et al* "Local Recurrence of Prostate Cancer after External Beam Radiation -Early Experience of Salvage Therapy Using High Intensity Focused Ultrasound." *Abstract. Uroweb,* March 17, 2005. www.uroweb.nl/index.

Scardino, Peter & Kelman, Judith. *The Prostate Book.* Avery (Penguin Group) Publication, New York, 2005.

Stanford, Janet *et al.* "Urinary and Sexual Function after Radical Prostatectomy for Clinically Localized Prostate Cancer." *Journal of the American Medical Association,* Vol. 283, No. 1, January 19, 2000: 354 - 360.

Steuber, T *et al.* "Transition Zone Cancers Undermine the Predictive Accuracy of Partin Table Stage Predictions." *The Journal of Urology,* Vol. 173 (3), March 2005: 737 – 741.

Strum, Stephen & Pogliano, Donna. *A Primer on Prostate Cancer – The Empowered Patient Guide.* The Life extensions Foundations, Florida, 2005

Stuart, Michael E. *et al.* "Cancer of the Prostate." *Journal of the American Medical Association,* Vol. 268, No. 22, December 9, 1992: 3197 - 3198.

Tomita, K *et al.* "Is Radical Prostatectomy Useful for Localized Prostatic Cancer Patients More than 71 Years Old?" *Abstract Uroweb,* March 17, 2005. www.uroweb.nl/index.

Walsh, Patrick. "Prostate Cancer Kills: Strategy to Reduce Deaths." *The Journal of Urology*, Vol. 44, No. 4, October 1994.

Walsh, Patrick & Worthington, Janet. *Guide to Surviving Prostate Cancer.* Warner Books, New York, 2001.

"Cryotherapy & High Intensity Focused Ultrasound." *The Prostate Cancer Research Institute.* February 2004, www.prostate-cancer.org.

"Questions to ask about prostate cancer." Canadian Cancer Society, November 3, 2003 - www.cancer.ca/ccs.

"What's New in Prostate Cancer and Treatment." American Cancer Society. May 2005, www.cancer.org/docroot/CRI/content/CRI/.

"HIFU with Ablatherm now Available in Canada for Patients with Prostate Cancer." April 2005. www.edap-hifu.com/.

"High Intensity Frequency Ultrasound (HIFU)." National Institute for Health and Clinical Excellence (NICE), March 2005. www.cancerhelp.org.uk.

Vancouver Prostate & Awareness Support Group. Notes from Lectures by Urologists & Oncologists, 2003 – 2005.

Chapter 8

Auerbach, Stephen. "The Treatment of Erectile Dysfunction." Prostate Cancer Research Institute, *Insights Newsletter,* August 2005, www.prostate-cancer.org/.

Auld, Brewer & Brock, Gerald. "Sexuality and Erectile Dysfunction: Results of a National Survey." *The Journal of Sexual & Reproductive Medicine,* Vol. 2, No. 2, Summer 2002: 50-54.

Brock, Gerald *et al.* "Safety and Efficacy of Vardenafil for Treatment of Men with Erectile Dysfunction." *The Journal of Urology*, Vol. 170 (4), October 2003: 1278 - 1283.

Burnett, Arthur L. "Erectile Dysfunction Following Radical Prostatectomy." *Journal of the American Medical Association,* Vol. 293, No. 21, June 1, 2005: 2648 - 2653.

Dr. Carter's Letter "Restoring Erections: Erectile Dysfunction & Viagra." *Johns Hopkins Bulletin,* 2003. www.prostatebulletin.com/.

Casey, Richard. "Testosterone Replacement Therapy." *The Journal of Sexual & Reproductive Medicine,* Vol. 3, No. 3, Autumn 2003.

Casey, Richard. Position Statement: "Sexuality Education: Counselling for the Primary Care Physician." *The Journal of Sexual & Reproductive Medicine,* Vol. 2, No. 1, Spring 2002.

Fleshner, Neil *et al.* "Evidence for Contamination of Herbal Erectile Dysfunction Products with Phosphodiesterase Type 5 Inhibitors." *The Journal of Urology,* Vol. 174, August 2005: 636 – 641.

Gaylis, Franklin *et al.* "Prostate Cancer in Men Using Testosterone Supplementation." *The Journal of Urology,* Vol. 174 (2), August 2005: 534 - 538.

Goldstein, Irwin *et al.* "Oral Sildenafil in the Treatment of Erectile Dysfunction." *New England Journal of Medicine,* Vol. 338, No. 20, May 1998: 1397 - 1404.

Greenstein, Alexander *et al.* "Does Sildenafil Combined with Testosterone Gel Improve Erectile Dysfunction in Hypogonadal Men in whom Testosterone Supplement Therapy Alone Failed?" *The Journal of Urology,* Vol. 173 (2), February 2005: 530-532.

Hatzichristou, D *et al.* "Effect of Tadalafil on Sexual Timing Behaviour Patterns in Men with Erectile Dysfunction: Integrated Analysis of Randomized, Placebo Controlled Trials." *The Journal of Urology,* Vol. 174, October 2005: 1356 – 1359.

Hong, Bumsik *et al.* "A Double Blind Crossover Study of Korean Ginseng in Patients with ED: A Preliminary Report." *The Journal of Urology,* Vol. 168, November 2002: 2070 - 2073.

Jiang, H *et al.* "Efficacy and safety of PGE1 cream in the Treatment of Erectile Dysfunction." Urology, Peking's University People's Hospital. *PubMed,* April 2003. www.ncbi.nlm.nih.gov/.

Kim, Edward *et al.* "Bilateral Nerve Graft during Radical Retropubic Prostatectomy: 1-Year Follow up." *The Journal of Urology,* Vol. 165 (6), June 2001: 1950 – 1956.

Kundu, Shilajit *et al.* "Potency, Continence and Complications in 3,477 Consecutive Radical Retrobubic Prostatectomies." *The Journal of Urology,* Vol. 172, December 2004: 2227 - 2231.

Matthew, Andrew *et al.* "Sexual Dysfunction after Radical Prostatectomy: Prevalence, Treatments, Restricted Use of Treatments and Distress." *The Journal of Urology*, Vol. 174, December 2005: 2105 – 2110.

Merrick, G.S. *et al.* "Erectile Dysfunction after Prostate Brachytherapy." *The Journal of Urology*, Vol. 175, March 2006: 959 – 960.

Munding, M.D *et al.* "Pilot study of Changes in Stretched Penile length 3 months after Radical Retropubic Prostatectomy." *PubMed*, 2001, www.ncbi.nlm.nih.gov/.

O'Leary, Michael *et al.* "Self-esteem, Confidence and Relationship Satisfaction of Men with Erectile Dysfunction Treated with Sildenafil Citrate: A Multicenter, Randomized, Parallel Group, Double-Blind, Placebo Controlled Study in the United States." *The Journal of Urology*, Vol. 175, March 2006: 1058 – 1062.

Parsons, Kellog J *et al.* "Serum Testosterone and the Risk of Prostate Cancer: Potential Implications for Testosterone Therapy." *Cancer Epidemiology Biomarkers & Prevention.* Vol. 14, September 2005: 2257 – 2260.

Rabbani, Farhang *et al.* "Factors Predicting Recovery of Erections after Radical Prostatectomy." *The Journal of Urology*, Vol. 164 (6), December 2000: 1929 - 1934.

Savoie, M *et al.* "A prospective study measuring Penile Length in men treated with Radical Prostatectomy." 2003. *PubMed.* www.ncbi.nlm.nih.gov/.

Scardino, Peter Judith. *The Prostate Book.* Avery (Penguin Group) Publication, New York, 2005.

Seftel, Allen et al. "The Efficacy and safety of Tadalafil in the United States and Puerto Rican Men with Erectile Dysfunction." Vol. 172, *The Journal of Urology*, August 2004: 652 - 657.

Severi, Gianluca et al. "Circulating Steroid Hormones and the Risk of Prostate Cancer." *Cancer Epidemiology Biomarkers & Prevention,* Vol. 15, January 2006: 86 – 91.

Shabsigh, R. et al. "Health Issues of Men: Prevalence and Correlates of Erectile Dysfunction." *The Journal of Urology,* Vol. 174, August 2005: 662 – 667.

Strum, Stephen & Pogliano, Donna. *A Primer on Prostate Cancer – The Empowered Patient Guide.* The Life Extensions Foundation, Florida, 2005.

The Male Health Centres: "Erectile Dysfunction" at www.malehealth.com.

Walsh, Patrick & Worthington, Janet. *Guide to Surviving Prostate Cancer.* Warner Books, 2001.

Vancouver Prostate & Awareness Support Group. Notes from Lectures by Urologists & Oncologists, 2003 – 2005.

Chapter 9

Albertsen, Peter *et al.* "20-Year Outcomes Following Conservative Management of Clinically Localized Prostate Cancer." *Journal of the American Medical Association,* Vol. 293, No. 17, May 4, 2005: 2095 - 2101.

Bill-Axelson, Anna *et al.* "Radical Prostatectomy versus Watchful Waiting in early Prostate Cancer." *New England J. Medicine,* Vol. 352, No. 19, May 12, 2005: 1977 - 1984.

Blasko, John & Wallner, Kent. *Prostate Brachytherapy.* Smart Medicine Press, Seattle, Washington, 1997.

Cadeddu, Jeffery *et al.* "Long-term Results of Radiation Therapy for Prostate Cancer Recurrence following Radical Prostatectomy." *The Journal of Urology,* Vol. 159 (1), January 1998: 173 – 177.

Catalona, William *et al.* "Cancer Recurrence and Survival Rates after Anatomic Radical Retropubic Prostatectomy for Prostate: Intermediate-Term Results." *The Journal of Urology,* Vol. 160 (6-II), December 1998: 2428 - 2434.

Catalona, William. "Recent Studies Raise Questions About Effectiveness of Radioactive Seed Implantation." Winter 2003. www.drcatalona.com/quest/.

Chaiken, Lisa *et al.* "Targeting for Cure: Intensity Modulated Radiation Therapy." Prostate Cancer Research Institute, *Insights Newsletter,* Vol. 7, No. 4, August 2004.

Chaudhary, Unzair *et al.* "Secondary hormonal manipulations in the management of advanced prostate cancer." *The Canadian Journal of Urology,* Vol. 12 (3), June 2005: 2666-2674.

Deger, S *et al.* "High Dose Rate Brachytherapy with Conformal Radiation Therapy for localized Prostate Cancer." European Urology, *PubMed,* April 2005 - www.ncbi.nih.gov/.

Gejerman, Glen. "Intensity Modulated Radiation Therapy." *Insights Newsletter,* Prostate Cancer Research Institute, Vol. 3, No. 1, April 2000.

Gleave, Martin *et al.* "Randomized Comparative Study of 3 versus 8 Month Neoadjuvant Hormonal Therapy before Radical Prostatectomy: Biochemical and Pathological Effects." *The Journal of Urology,* Vol. 166 (2), August 2001: 500 – 507.

Gleave, Martin *et al.* "Biochemical and Pathological Effects of 8 Months of Neoadjuvant Androgen Withdrawal Therapy before Radical Prostatectomy in Patients with Clinically Confined Prostate Cancer." *The Journal of Urology,* Vol. 155 (1), January 1996: 213 – 219.

Grimm, Peter *et al.* "Prostate Seed Implantation for Prostate Cancer." Prostate Cancer Research Institute, *Insights Newsletter,* Vol. 6, No. 8, November 2003.

Hall, Celia. "Vaccine for Cervical Cancer." *Medical Editor,* July, 2005. www.telegraph.co.uk.

Holmberg, L *et al.* "A Randomized Trial comparing Radical Prostatectomy with Watchful Waiting in Early Prostate Cancer. *New England Journal of Medicine,* Vol. 347, September 12, 2002: 781 – 789.

Johansson, Jan-Erik *et al.* "Natural History of Early, Localized Prostate Cancer." *Journal of the American Medical Association,* Vol. 291, No. 22, June 9, 2004: 2713 - 2719.

Liu, M *et al.* "Urinary Incontinence in Prostate Cancer Patients Treated with External Beam Radiation." *Radiotherapy Oncology*, February 2005:197 - 2001 - www.ncbi.nlm.nih.gov/.

Lukka, Himu *et al.* "Prostate cancer Radiotherapy 2002 - the way forward." *The Canadian Journal of Urology,* Vol. 12, No. 1, February 2005: 2521 - 2531.

Mabjeesh, N *et al.* "Sexual Function after Permanent Iodine 125 Brachytherapy for Prostate Cancer." *International Journal of Impotence Research,* Vol. 17, October 2004: 96 – 101.

McKenzie, Michael. "Radiation Therapy for Prostate Cancer." B.C. Cancer Agency Library File, 1995.

Our Voice – Living with Prostate Cancer in Canada. Spring, Summer, Fall, & Winter Issues, 1998 – 2004

Our Voice (New Edition) – Living with Prostate Cancer in Canada. Vols. 1 & 2, Nos. 1& 2, Summer & Fall 2005.

Pether, Michael *et al.* "Intermittent Androgen Suppression in Prostate Cancer: an Update of the Vancouver Experience." *The Canadian Journal of Urology*, Vol. 10 (2), April, 2003: 1809 - 1814.

Pound, Charles *et al.* "Natural History of Progression after PSA Elevation following Radical Prostatectomy." *Journal of the American Medical Association,* Vol. 281, No. 17, May 1999: 1591 – 1597.

Prostate Cancer - A Booklet for Patients. Canadian Prostate Cancer Network. Lakefield, Ontario, 2003.

Scardino, Peter & Kelman, Judith. *The Prostate Book.* Avery (Penguin Group) Publication, New York, 2005.

Shahinian, Vahakn *et al.* "Risk of Fracture after Androgen Deprivation for Prostate Cancer." *New England J. Medicine,* Vol. 352, No. 2, January 13, 2005: 154 - 164.

Sharifi, Nima *et al.* "Androgen Deprivation Therapy for Prostate Cancer." *JAMA,* Vol. 294, No. 2, July 13, 2005: 238 - 244.

Shen, Samson *et al.* "Ultrasensitive Serum Prostate Specific Antigen Nadir Accurately Predicts the Risk of Early Relapse after Radical Prostatectomy." *The Journal of Urology,* Vol. 173 (3), March 2005: 777-780.

Sherar, Micheal *et al.* "Interstitial Microwave Thermal Therapy for Prostate Cancer: Method of Treatment and Results of Phase 1/11 Trial." *The Journal of Urology,* Vol. 166 (5), November 2001: 1707 – 1714.

Stephenson, Andrew *et al.* "Salvage Radiotherapy for Recurrent Prostate Cancer after Radical Prostatectomy." *Journal of the American Medical Association,* Vol. 291, No. 11, March 17, 2004: 1325 - 1332.

Strom, Sara *et al.* "Obesity, Weight Gain, and Risk of Biochemical Failure among Prostate Cancer patients following Prostatectomy." *Clinical Cancer Research,* Vol. 11, October 2005: 6889 – 6894.

Strum, Stephen & Pogliano, Donna. *A Primer on Prostate Cancer – The Empowered Patient Guide.* The Life Extension Foundation, Florida, 2005.

Tannock, Ian *et al.* "Docetaxel plus Prednistone or Mitoxanthrone plus Prednistone for Advanced Cancer." *New England Journal of Medicine,* Vol. 351, No. 15, October 7, 2004: 1502 - 1512.

Tyldesley, Scott. Discussion with Radiation Oncologist Tyldesley and Author, B.C. Cancer Agency, 2005.

Walsh, Patrick & Worthington, Janet. *Guide to Surviving Prostate Cancer.* Warner Books, New York, 2001.

"High Cholesterol levels accelerate the Growth of Prostate Cancer." Children's Hospital, Boston. March 2005. www.sciencedaily.com.

"B.C. Cancer Agency launches first-of-its- kind prostate cancer study in Western Canada." July 13, 2005. www.bccancer.bc.ca.

"ProstaScint May Detect Recurrent Prostate Cancer Earlier." American Cancer Society, July 2001. www.cancer.org/docroot/.

Dr. Catalona's Website (www.catalona.com/quest/)

"New Results for Postoperative Radiotherapy", Summer 2004.

"Intensity Modulated Radiation Therapy." Prostate Cancer Research Institute, August 2003, www.prostate-cancer.org/education/.

"Vaccine Slows PSA Increase in Hormone Refractory Prostate Cancer." 2005. http:/patient.cancerconsultants.com.

Dr. Catalona's Website (www.catalona.com/quest/)

"Hormonal Therapy Explained." Winter 2003.

Vancouver Prostate & Awareness Support Group. Notes from lectures by Oncologists, 2003 – 2005.

Chapter 10

Canadian Cancer Society: www.cancer.ca.

American Cancer Society: www.cancer.org.

Prostate Cancer Research Institute: www.prostate-cancer.org.

Prostate Support Group – Us Too: www.ustoo.com.

Canadian Prostate Health Council: www.canadian-prostate.com.

Canadian Prostate Cancer Network: www.cpcn.org.

Centre for Integrated Healing: www.healing.bc.ca.

Centre for Integrated Healing. *An Introduction to Integrated Healing.* Suite 200, 1330 W. 8 th Ave., Vancouver, B.C., March 2005.

Phillips, Robert, H. *Coping With Prostate Cancer.* Avery Publication Co., New York, 1994.

"People Living with Cancer Coping." January 2005, www.plwc.org/.

"Coping: Talking to Your Children…Your Teenagers…Your Spouse or Partner about Cancer." January 2005. www.plwc.org/plwc/.

The Canadian Prostate Health Council Pamphlets, Dorval, Quebec, H9R 4P8, 1997.

Chapter 11

Buettner, Dan. "The Secrets of Long Life." *National Geographic Magazine,* November 2005.

Chopra, Deepak. *Ageless Body, Timeless Mind.* Harmony Books, New York, 1993.

Fradet, Yves *et al.* "uPM3, a new Molecular Urine Test for the Detection of Prostate Cancer." *Urology*, Vol. 64, No. 2, August 2004: 311 – 316.

Giovannucci, E.L *et al.* "A Prospective Study of Physical Activity and Incident and Fatal Prostate Cancer." *PubMed,* May 9, 2005.

Kopek, Jacek *et al.* "Screening with Prostate Specific Antigen and Metastatic Prostate Cancer Risk: A Population Based Case-Controlled Study." *The Journal of Urology*, Vol. 174 (2), August 2005: 475 – 499.

McKenzie, D.C. "The Importance of Exercise in Prostate Cancer Therapy." Lecture at the Vancouver Prostate Support & Awareness Group, November 2005.

Thompson, Ian *et al.* "Prevalence of Prostate Cancer among Men with a Prostate-Specific Antigen Level of less than or equal to 4.o ng/ml." *New England Journal of Medicine*, Vol. 350, No. 22, May, 2004: 2239 – 2246.

Walsh, Patrick & Worthington, Janet. *Guide to Surviving Prostate Cancer.* Warner Books, New York, 2001.

Canadian Cancer Society: www.cancer.ca.

The Canadian Prostate Health Council: www.canadian-prostate.com.

National Cancer Institute of Canada: www.nci.cancer.ca.

Canadian Urological Association: www.cua.org/.

American Urological Association: www.auanet.org/.

Canadian Prostate Cancer Network: www.cpcn.org.

Canadian Association of Provincial Cancer Agencies: www.capca.ca.

Centre for Integrated Healing: www.healing.bc.ca.

Information on Frauds, Fads and Myths: www.quackwatch.org.